Advances in Anatomy, Embryology and Cell Biology
Ergebnisse der Anatomie und Entwicklungsgeschichte
Revues d'anatomie et de morphologie expérimentale
Springer-Verlag Berlin Heidelberg New York

This journal publishes reviews and critical articles covering the entire field of normal anatomy (cytology, histology, cyto- and histochemistry, electron microscopy, macroscopy, experimental morphology and embryology and comparative anatomy). Papers dealing with anthropology and clinical morphology will also be accepted with the aim of encouraging co-operation between anatomy and related disciplines.

Papers, which may be in English, French or German, are normally commissioned, but original papers and communications may be submitted and will be considered so long as they deal with a subject comprehensively and meet the requirements of the Ergebnisse.

For speed of publication and breadth of distribution, this journal appears in single issues which can be purchased separately; 6 issues constitute one volume.

It is a fundamental condition that manuscripts submitted should not have been published elsewhere, in this or any other country, and the author must undertake not to publish elsewhere at a later date.

25 copies of each paper are supplied free of charge.

Les résultats publient des sommaires et des articles critiques concernant l'ensemble du domaine de l'anatomie normale (cytologie, histologie, cyto et histochimie, microscopie électronique, macroscopie, morphologie expérimentale, embryologie et anatomie comparée. Seront publiés en outre les articles traitant de l'anthropologie et de la morphologie clinique, en vue d'encourager la collaboration entre l'anatomie et les disciplines voisines.

Seront publiés en priorité les articles expressément demandés nous tiendrons toutefois compte des articles qui nous seront envoyés dans la mesure où ils traitent d'un sujet dans son ensemble et correspondent aux standards des «Résultats». Les publications seront faites en langues anglaise, allemande et française.

Dans l'intérêt d'une publication rapide et d'une large diffusion les travaux publiés paraitront dans des cahiers individuels, diffusés séparément: 6 cahiers forment un volume.

En principe, seuls les manuscrits qui n'ont encore été publiés ni dans le pays d'origine ni à l'étranger peuvent nous être soumis. L'auteur d'engage en outre à ne pas les publier ailleurs ultérieurement.

Les auteurs recevront 25 exemplaires gratuits de leur publication.

Die Ergebnisse dienen der Veröffentlichung zusammenfassender und kritischer Artikel aus dem Gesamtgebiet der normalen Anatomie (Cytologie, Histologie, Cyto- und Histochemie, Elektronenmikroskopie, Makroskopie, experimentelle Morphologie und Embryologie und vergleichende Anatomie). Aufgenommen werden ferner Arbeiten anthropologischen und morphologisch-klinischen Inhaltes, mit dem Ziel, die Zusammenarbeit zwischen Anatomie und Nachbardisziplinen zu fördern.

Zur Veröffentlichung gelangen in erster Linie angeforderte Manuskripte, jedoch werden auch eingesandte Arbeiten und Orginalmitteilungen berücksichtigt, sofern sie ein Gebiet umfassend abhandeln und den Anforderungen der ,,Ergebnisse" genügen. Die Veröffentlichungen erfolgen in englischer, deutscher und französicher Sprache.

Die Arbeiten erscheinen im Interesse einer raschen Veröffentlichung und einer weiten Verbreitung als einzeln berechnete Hefte; je 6 Hefte bilden einen Band.

Grundsätzlich dürfen nur Manuskripte eingesandt werden, die vorher weder im Inland noch im Ausland veröffentlicht worden sind. Der Autor verpflichtet sich, sie auch nachträglich nicht an anderen Stellen zu publizieren.

Die Mitarbeiter erhalten von ihren Arbeiten zusammen 25 Freiexemplare.

Manuscripts should be addressed to/Envoyer les manucsrits à/Manuskripte sind zu senden an:

Prof. Dr. A. BRODAL, Universitetet i Oslo, Anatomisk Institutt, Karl Johans Gate 47 (Domus Media), Oslo 1/Norwegen

Prof. W. HILD, Department of Anatomy. The University of Texas Medical Branch, Galveston, Texas 77550 (USA)

Prof. Dr. J. van LIMBORGH, Universiteit van Amsterdam, Anatomisch-Embryologisch Laboratorium, Amsterdam-O/Holland, Mauritskade 61

Prof. Dr. R. ORTMANN, Anatomisches Institut der Universität, D-5000 Köln-Lindenthal, Lindenburg

Prof. Dr. T. H. SCHIEBLER, Anatomisches Institut der Universität, Koellikerstraße 6, D-8700 Würzburg

Prof. Dr. G. TÖNDURY, Direktion der Anatomie, Gloriastraße 19, CH-8006 Zürich

Prof. Dr. E. WOLFF, Collège de France, Laboratoire d'Embryologie Expérimentale, 49 bis Avenue de la belle Gabrielle, Nogent-sur-Marne 94/France

Advances in Anatomy, Embryology and Cell Biology
Ergebnisse der Anatomie und Entwicklungsgeschichte
Revues d'anatomie et de morphologie expérimentale

47 · 4

Editors
A. Brodal, Oslo · W. Hild, Galveston · J. van Limborgh, Amsterdam
R. Ortmann, Köln · T. H. Schiebler, Würzburg · G. Töndury, Zürich · E. Wolff, Paris

Finn-Mogens Šmejda Haug

Heavy Metals in the Brain

A Light Microscope Study of the Rat with Timm's Sulphide
Silver Method. Methodological Considerations and Cytological
and Regional Staining Patterns

With 40 Figures

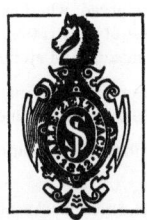

Springer-Verlag Berlin Heidelberg New York 1973

Dr. Finn-Mogens Šmejda Haug
Anatomical Institute
University of Oslo
Karl Johansgt. 47, Oslo 1
Norway

The present manuscript has been referred to previously under the title: Selective staining of central nervous structures with Timm's sulphide silver method for heavy metals. A light microscope study in the rat.

ISBN 978-3-540-06213-4   ISBN 978-3-642-51585-9 (eBook)
DOI 10.1007/978-3-642-51585-9

This work is subject to copyright. All rights are reserved, whether the whole or part of the material is concerned, specifically those of translation, reprinting, re-use of illustrations, broadcasting, reproduction by photocopying machine or similar means, and storage in data banks.

Under § 54 of the German Copyright Law where copies are made for other than private use, a fee is payable to the publisher, the amount of the fee to be determined by agreement with the publisher.

© by Springer-Verlag Berlin·Heidelberg 1973. Library of Congress Catalog Card Number 73-11599

The use of general descriptive names, trade names, trade marks, etc. in this publication, even if the former are not especially identified, is not to be taken as a sign that such names, as understood by the Trade Marks and Merchandise Marks Act, may accordingly be used freely by anyone.

Contents

Abbreviations Used in Low Power Micrographs 7

I. Introduction 9

II. Material and Methods 10
    A. Sulphide Treatment, Sectioning and Postfixation 10
    B. Staining of Sections ("Physical Development") 11
    C. Preparation of Paraffin Material 12
    D. Photography of Sections 13

III. Observations 13
    A. Temporal Course of the Development 13
    B. General Distribution of the Stain in Grey and White Matter 15
        1. Neuropil 16
            a) Telencephalon 16, b) Brain Stem 18 16
        2. Neuronal Perikarya 18
        3. Neuroglia and Vessels 21
            a) Glial Cells 21, b) Ependyma and Choroid Plexus 25, c) Vessels 25 . . . 21
        4. Axons and Myelin 25
    C. Regional Staining Patterns 27
        1. Telencephalon 27
        2. Diencephalon 35
        3. Mesencephalon 39
        4. Pons and Medulla Oblongata 41
        5. Cerebellum 43
        6. Spinal Cord 43

IV. Discussion 48
    A. The Sulphide Silver Method 48
    B. Variations in the Results 50
    C. Chemical Interpretation of the Staining 51
    D. The Cellular Localization of the Stain 55
        1. Neuronal Perikarya 56
        2. Neuroglia 56
        3. Neuropil 58
            a) Telencephalon 58, b) Brain Stem, Cerebellum and Spinal Cord 59 58
    E. Timm Staining of Paraffin Sections 59
    F. Concluding Remarks 60
        1. The Morphological Significance of the Regional Staining Patterns 60
        2. Possible Functional Implications of the Staining 60

V. Summary and Conclusions 62

Acknowledgements 63

References 64

Subject Index 70

Abbreviations Used in Low Power Micrographs

AC	commissura anterior		el	area entorhinalis, pars lateralis
C	cingulum		em	area entorhinalis, pars medialis
CC	corpus callosum		ep	nucleus entopeduncularis
CI	capsula interna		fd	fascia dentata
CH	commissura habenularis		gp	globus pallidus
CP	commissura posterior		hal	nucleus habenularis lateralis
DB	nucleus and tractus diagonalis Broca		ham	nucleus habenularis medialis
F	fornix		harc	nucleus arcuatus hypothalami
FI	fimbria		hl	area hypothalamica lateralis
FR	fasciculus retroflexus		hpv	nucleus paraventricularis hypo-thalami
LM	lemniscus medialis			
LME	lamina medullaris externa (thalami)		hsc	nucleus suprachiasmaticus hypo-thalami
LOT	tractus olfactorius lateralis			
OC	chiasma opticum		hso	nucleus supraopticus hypothalami
OT	tractus opticus		hvm	nucleus ventromedialis hypothalami
P	pedunculus cerebri		hy	hypothalamus
PCM	pedunculus cerebellaris medius		im	insula Calleja Magna
PCS	pedunculus cerebellaris superior		in	nucleus interstitialis (Cajal)
PCI	pedunculus cerebellaris inferior		ip	nucleus interpeduncularis
PD	psalterium dorsale		lf	lamina fibrillorum of olfactory bulb
SM	stria medullaris		lg	lamina glomerulosa of olfactory bulb
ST	stria terminalis		ll	nuclei leminisci lateralis
T	fasciculus mammillothalamicus		lot	nucleus tractus olfactorius lateralis
W	white matter of the olfactory bulb		lpe	lamina plexiformis externa of olfactory bulb
a	amygdala			
aaa	area amygdaloidea anterior		m	corpus mammillare
acc	nucleus accumbens septi		mes	mesencephalon
avt	area ventralis tegmenti		ni	substantia nigra
bo	bulbus olfactorius		np	pontine nuclei
boa	bulbus olfactorius accessorius		oa	nucleus olfactorius anterior
cd	nucleus cochlearis dorsalis		oi	oliva inferior
cg	central gray matter of the mesencephalon		os	oliva superior
			ot	tuberculum olfactorium
cgld	corpus geniculatum laterale, dorsal nucleus		p	posterior column nuclei
			pi	corpus pineale
cglv	corpus geniculatum laterale, ventral nucleus		pl	plexus chorioideus
			pol	regio preoptica lateralis
cgm	corpus geniculatum mediale		ps	presubiculum
cn	cerebellar nuclei		pt	pretectal region (see text p. 39)
co	locus coeruleus		pyr	pyriform cortex
coll i	colliculus inferior		r	nucleus ruber
coll s	colliculus superior		rf	reticular formation
comm	nucleus commissuralis		rt	nucleus reticularis tegmenti pontis
cp	nucleus caudatus-putamen		s	septal area
cs	nucleus centralis superior		sl	nucleus septi lateralis
ct	nucleus of corpus trapezoideum		sm	nucleus septi medialis
cv	nucleus cochlearis ventralis		st	nucleus proprius striae terminalis
dt	nucleus dorsalis tegmenti		subt	nucleus subthalamicus

sol	nucleus tractus solitarius	*III*	region of the occulomotor nucleus
t	thalamus	*V*	nucleus motorius nervi trigemini
tad	nucleus anterior dorsalis thalami	*Vnm*	nucleus mesencephalicus nervi
tam	nucleus anterior medialis thalami		trigemini
tav	nucleus anterior ventralis thalami	*Vp*	nucleus principalis nervi trigemini
tl	nucleus lateralis thalami	*Vs*	nucleus tractus spinalis nervi
tm	nucleus dorsomedialis thalami		trigemini
tpf	nucleus parafascicularis thalami	*Vr*	root of trigeminal nerve
tr	nucleus reticularis thalami	*VII*	nucleus nervi facialis
tv	nucleus ventralis thalami	*VIIg*	genu nervi facialis
v	nucleus vestibularis superior and	*VIIr*	facial root-fibres
	medialis	*X*	nucleus motorius dorsalis nervi vagi
vl	nucleus vestibularis lateralis	*XII*	nucleus nervi hypoglossi
vs	nucleus vestibularis spinalis	*3*	third ventricle
vt	nucleus ventralis tegmenti	*4*	fourth ventricle
	(von Gudden)	*29b*	cingulate cortex
zi	zona incerta	*29c*	cingulate cortex

I. Introduction

The importance of transition metals and group IIb metals in biological reactions is becoming increasingly clear. Such metals form an integral part of the structure of many enzymes and non-enzymic proteins and also feature in more reversible interactions between metal ions and large or small biological molecules (Johnson and Seven, 1961). As discussed at the end of this paper, chemical analyses have shown the presence of these metals in the central nervous system and some hypotheses have been advanced concerning their role in more specific nervous activities such as synaptic processes. In order to define more precisely the role of these trace metals it is clearly necessary to investigate their regional and cytological distribution, as may be achieved by the use of histochemical methods.

Some of the earliest neurohistochemical studies were concerned with trace metals, especially iron, in the brain (Spatz, 1922). Later reports on the localization of trace metals have been comparatively few, except as regards the hippocampal region.

Maske's report (1955) that intravital injections of the coloured chelating agent, dithizone, revealed an accumulation of zinc within the hippocampus, prompted a series of investigations by Fleischhauer and Horstmann (1957), Timm (1958a), McLardy (1960, 1962, 1963, 1964), von Euler (1962), and others, in which the intravital dithizone method or Timm's sulphide silver method was used. As a result, particularly intense staining was found to correspond to the zones receiving mossy fibre terminals (Cajal, 1911; Blackstad et al., 1970). Von Euler (1962), in particular, presented evidence that the stain is localized to the mossy fibre boutons, that it is due to the presence of zinc and that the metal is necessary for the transmission of impulses here. Electron microscopy (Haug, 1967; Ibata and Otsuka, 1969) and chemical analyses (Hu and Friede, 1968) have confirmed that the staining is confined to the boutons and, in all likelihood, is due to the presence of zinc.

The uniquely intense staining of the mossy fibre system seems to have overshadowed the fact that there is staining also of other structures with dithizone and with Timm's method. Timm (1961) briefly mentions that in addition to the staining of somata there is in many parts of the brain a variegated staining of the neuropil which he assumes to be of great importance. He offers no further interpretation of this staining and gives few illustrations. McLardy (1964) describes a strong sulphide silver staining in the neuropil of the subiculum, interpreted as a second hippocampal zinc-rich system. He also comments on a widespread background brownness in various parts of the telencephalon, which is visible in his photomicrographs of Timm stained sections, and suggests that this also reflects staining of synapses (McLardy, 1963).

The intriguing possibility that the zinc-containing mossy fibre boutons may have counterparts in several other synaptic systems, invites further investigations. Light microscope analyses of the regional and cytological distribution of the stain in various parts of the nervous system are among the first logical steps in such an investigation.

It is the purpose of the present study:

1. To describe slight modifications of the sulphide silver method that favour a particularly strong staining of the central nervous system.

2. To give a survey of the highly differentiated pattern which is then revealed, and

3. To discuss its possible significance from a histochemical point of view.

It is emphasized that the present report can only give an introductory survey of the staining pattern and that, in general, no attempt will be made to relate the staining pattern fully to existing knowledge of structure, connexions and chemoarchitecture of individual regions of the brain.

II. Material and Methods

Young adult albino rats (Wistar strain) of both sexes were used.

During the past five years, several hundred rat brains have been processed for various purposes, using the method described below. As a rule, three or four parallel series were made from each brain, two being stained according to the sulphide silver method and the others using conventional histological methods as needed.

For the purpose of the present report, nine additional brains were processed with particular care to avoid any deformation in the final sections. For each brain, all the sections were mounted to form three parallel frontal, sagittal, or horizontal series. The two series were sulphide silver stained and one was stained with thionine.

Sections were also selected from other series in order to illustrate various cytological features.

Several modifications of the sulphide silver method of Timm have been described (Timm, 1958b; Voigt, 1951, 1959; Brunk et al., 1968; and others). The principal steps of the method are sulphide-precipitation of metals in the tissue followed by a so-called physical development. During the latter stage the metal sulphides catalyze reduction of silver ions by hydroquinone or other reducing agents. Brunk and Sköld (1967) showed that an artefactual distribution of precipitate may result from paraffin embedding (an observation also made in the present study). As a consequence, cryostat sections were used throughout this study—with one exception that will be discussed later. The cryostat procedures described in this paper have given consistent results within the forebrain of several hundred rats (see also p. 50). Details of the staining within the brain stem were mainly studied in four frontal series, and the spinal cord was examined in only one animal. The present paper primarily reports results obtained with the standardized cryostat modification described below, the limits within which the procedures may be varied without significantly affecting the final result having been determined in separate experiments. Since a few illustrations of older paraffin material are included, the corresponding procedures are also briefly described.

A. Sulphide Treatment, Sectioning and Postfixation

The animals are anaesthetized with ether and Nembutal and perfused through the left ventricle with a solution of 11.7 g Na_2S and 11.9 g $NaH_2PO_4 \cdot H_2O$ per 1 000 ml H_2O. (Sodium sulphide is hygroscopic and is oxidized by air; hence a fresh supply should be used.) The solution will be clear and colourless and have a pH of 7.3–7.4[1]. Perfusion is performed at

1 For practical reasons the solution was sometimes made up on the day before perfusion took place. It then acquired a yellow tinge overnight. This did not cause significant differences in the staining from cases where fresh solution was used—as specifically determined in separate experiments.

room temperature from a height of 100–110 centimetres, using a 2.0 mm Wassermann canula and a transparent tubing from which air bubbles may be carefully excluded. The perfusion is considered successful when characterized by an immediate, rapid flow and resulting in strong muscular contractions together with paling of skin, eyes and viscera within 20 seconds. A strong greyish to green tint of eyes, skin and viscera appears within approximately one minute, and the liver usually becomes almost black within less than 5 minutes. In some animals the darkening of viscera, particularly the liver, is less marked (but the staining pattern of the brain is normal). After 1 minute of rapid flow, the rate of perfusion may be reduced to 5–10 ml per minute as determined by an inserted drop chamber. Standard perfusion time is 20 minutes, during which 200–300 ml perfusate is usually consumed. When removed, the brains have the soft consistency of an unfixed brain, but show an even, greyish-green tinge.

The brains are quickly frozen with CO_2-gas and sectioned in a cryostat (Model Dittes Duspiva) at 2–40 microns; the sections are mounted on microscope slides by thawing. Several sections are mounted on each slide in serial order. After drying in air for 15 minutes to two hours, the sections are postfixed in 96 percent ethanol for 15 minutes, hydrated through an alcohol series and subsequently stained within 5–10 minutes. Several hours postfixation in alcohol causes a loss of part of the stain.

Frozen brains or sections may be stored for at least 3 days at $-25°$ C with negligible loss of stainability. The frozen brains are wrapped in plastic foil or kept in closed vials. Sections are stored in desiccated and sealed boxes.

To protect the experimenter from inhaling hydrogen sulphide all procedures involving sulphide solutions, including pH measurements, perfusion and dissection of the brains, should be carried out under a fully efficient hood. The animals may be placed on a wire grid above a sink which is continuously flushed with water, or above a container with a small amount of formaldehyde solution (which reacts with sulphide). The perfused bodies may be treated with formaldehyde before they are removed.

B. Staining of Sections ("Physical Development")

In order to obtain fair uniformity of staining, which is important when comparing sections from different brains or within large series from the same brain, slides may be processed in bulk. Ordinary histological utensils are used but should be chemically clean. Development is carried out in total darkness as suggested by Brunk et al. (1968) and at a fixed temperature of 24° C. If the temperature is raised to this point by a waterbath, it is important that the staining vessels is virtually submerged, so as to avoid a gradient of decreasing stain intensity towards the top of the slides. Furthermore, the slides should be evenly spaced in the staining rack.

It is necessary to investigate the effect of a wide range of staining times, since the degree of development which is best to bring out details in one structure may not be optimal for others in the same section (cp. section III-A, p. 13). One or more degrees of stain intensity suitable for the immediate object of study may then be chosen and adhered to for the preparation of further material. Despite the measure of standardization described, a given development time does not consistently produce the same degree of impregnation. Sample sections from each batch must, therefore, be briefly removed from the staining jar and inspected towards the end of the development. They should be compared *against a lighted background*, with a display of corresponding sections developed for increasing lengths of time. In our hands a useful standard series covering the full range of contrast was prepared by developing for 30, 40, 50, 60, 70, 80, and 90 minutes.

Stock Solutions

Citrate Buffer, 2 M. Citric acid · H_2O 25.5 g; tri-sodium citrate · $2H_2O$ 23.5 g; de-ionized water ad 100 ml. This buffer may be kept at room temperature for some days and is warmed gently before use to redissolve crystals. On dilution 1:10 the pH is approximately 4.0.

 ᶜ *Hydroquinone Solution.* Hydroquinone 5.67 g; de-ionized water ad 100 ml. This should be prepared not more than a few hours before use.

Gum Arabic Solution. Gum arabic (large pieces, not powder) 4 kg; de-ionized water ad 8 litres. Dissolution takes several days and must be aided by frequent stirring and digging into the sticky mass at the bottom of the container. A wide jar is, therefore, used. After about 10 days the solution is filtered through several layers of gauze, and divided between conveniently small polyethylene bottles for storage in a deep freeze, where it may be kept for several months. When removed from the deep freeze, it may be kept refrigerated, but should be discarded if not used within a week. Gum arabic is a natural product whose properties may vary. It was obtained by this author from Riedel de Hahn (Hannover) or Bie & Berntsen (Copenhagen). On dissolution it had a pH of 4.2 when occasionally measured.

Silver Nitrate Solution. Silver nitrate 8.5 g; de-ionized water 50 ml. The solution may be kept for several days if refrigerated and protected from light. It should be discarded if black grains of reduced silver are visible.

The Staining Solution. Gum arabic 60 ml; citrate buffer 10 ml; hydroquinone 30 ml; silver nitrate 0.5 ml. The final solution has a pH of 3.8–3.9; is 0.2 M in citrate; 0.15 M (1.7%) in hydroquinone; 5×10^{-3} M (0.085%) in silver nitrate, and approximately 30% in Gum arabic. The mixture of the first three solutions will keep for some hours but the complete developer should be used immediately. The developer decays more quickly when illuminated, but need not be protected from dimmed light during the 1–2 minutes it takes to stir in the silver nitrate and pour the solution into staining jars already filled with slides. Nor is the staining pattern qualitatively affected by occasional short inspections of sections during the staining, using moderate artificial or diffuse day light. During the staining the developer decays spontaneously and becomes greyish brown, but usually not quite impenetrable to light during the time required to produce strong staining of the sections. The speed of decay varies even if the developer is carefully prepared.

The staining is stopped by a thorough rinse in tap water for at least 5 minutes to remove the viscous developer. The sections are then dehydrated in alcohol, cleared briefly in xylene, and enclosed under cover slips with dammar resin. The stained sections may be left in formalin or alcohol over-night, but if left in xylene will bleach completely. Under cover glass the staining is usually quite stable, but some series bleach within months or even weeks. Parts of sections extending beyond the cover glass will bleach, presumably due to oxidation. Acids or aetheroleum cajeputi quickly bleach the stain. Thionine or hematoxylin may be used for counterstaining, but a certain bleaching of the sulphide silver stain may result even at a neutral pH. Acid solutions should not be used for differentiation or for lowering the pH of the staining solution. The sections should be differentiated in alcohol instead.

It has not proved possible to defer the sulphide treatment until after freezing and sectioning in order to allow alternating sections to be stained with Timm's method and other methods, with which sulphide might interfere. Nor may aldehyde fixation be used without precautions. However, the modification of Fink-Heimer's method described by Hjorth-Simonsen (1970) for cryostat sections of unfixed brains gives fairly satisfactory results on sulphide perfused material (Haug et al., 1971), and the original Nauta method may be similarly applied after formalin postfixation of the sections. The acetylcholinesterase pattern is also unaffected by the sulphide treatment.

C. Preparation of Paraffin Material

The animals were anaesthetized with ether and decapitated. The brains were dissected out and fixed in Carnoy's solution containing 1.2% Na_2S. After a fixation period of 24–48 hours the brains were stored for a few days more in absolute alcohol and embedded in paraffin by a routine procedure lasting for several days. Some brains were only briefly washed with absolute alcohol and then embedded in the course of 8 hours, using continuous agitation of the fluids, to which (including the paraffin) sulphide was added in some experiments. None of these experiments gave better results than the routine procedure.

Sections were cut, floated on water, stretched by heating and dried overnight at 37° C. They were then deparaffinized, hydrated and stained by physical development as described above.

D. Photography of Sections

Photomacrographs were taken on a conventional equipment (Leitz Aristophot with Leitz *Summar* or Zeiss *Luminar* lenses, a 30 watt tungsten light source, no filters) using 9 × 12 Kodak Ektapan or Plus X Pan cut-film. Photomicrographs were taken on various photomicroscopes using 36 mm Kodak Panatomic X or Adox KB 14 film; or 9 × 12 cm Plus X Pan or Ektapan cut film.

The high contrast between unstained and maximally stained structures is difficult to accommodate on photographic material so that sections with a degree of staining suitable for the specific structures to be demonstrated had to be selected from different series. The survey pictures in Figs. 19 to 38 are taken from one uniformly stained series, however. Each negative was exposed individually to give the best photographic result and, during enlargement, the prints were shadowed by hand if necessary to prevent over-exposure of the print in the darkest areas. The final prints resulting from these procedures, represent the relative staining densities of various areas satisfactorily in principle but only in a qualitative sense.

III. Observations

A. Temporal Course of the Development

The different brain structures stain in a sequence which is of interest both as a guide to optimal development and as an indication of the concentration of stainable substances within them.

Typically, a slight yellow tinge is visible macroscopically in the hippocampal mossy fibre areas and the neuropil in some other strongly reactive forebrain areas after 20 to 30 minutes. At higher magnifications, individual mossy fibre boutons are then faintly discernible, whereas many neuronal perikarya and glial cells already contain a black stain. At this early stage the stain in neuronal perikarya and certain glial cells (*1*, p. 21; *2*, p. 21) can thus be studied without interference from staining in the neuropil.

Continued development increases the staining of perikarya but above all that of the neuropil (p. 16). After 50 to 60 minutes, the hippocampal mossy fiber zones and individual giant boutons have turned black so that further development can contribute little more apparent density to these structures. Other parts of the neuropil stain more slowly and remain far paler even after the longest development time used. Thus, the more weakly reactive parts of the telencephalic neuropil such as fascia dentata (p. 34) require 40 to 50 minutes to become faintly stained and are still darkening between 70 and 90 minutes, differentiating into zones of widely varying density from unstained to dark brown. Similarly, many details of regional differentiation within the brain stem and spinal cord that are only faintly discernible at 60 minutes become conspicuous at 80 to 90 minutes. Weakly reactive glial processes (*3*, p. 21) in several fibre tracts require 70 to 90 minutes to become clearly visible.

Obviously the early strong granulation of perikarya and the homogeneous black staining of glial cells are obscured amidst reactive neuropil if development is continued, as are slight regional differences of the neuropil itself within very dark areas. It is important to note, however, that within both grey and white matter unstained structures are still conspicuous, showing that the method remains selective even at levels of development which originally were considered excessive.

Macroscopically, the sections after 50 to 60 minutes of development include areas stained light yellow, brown or black and give an over all impression of being

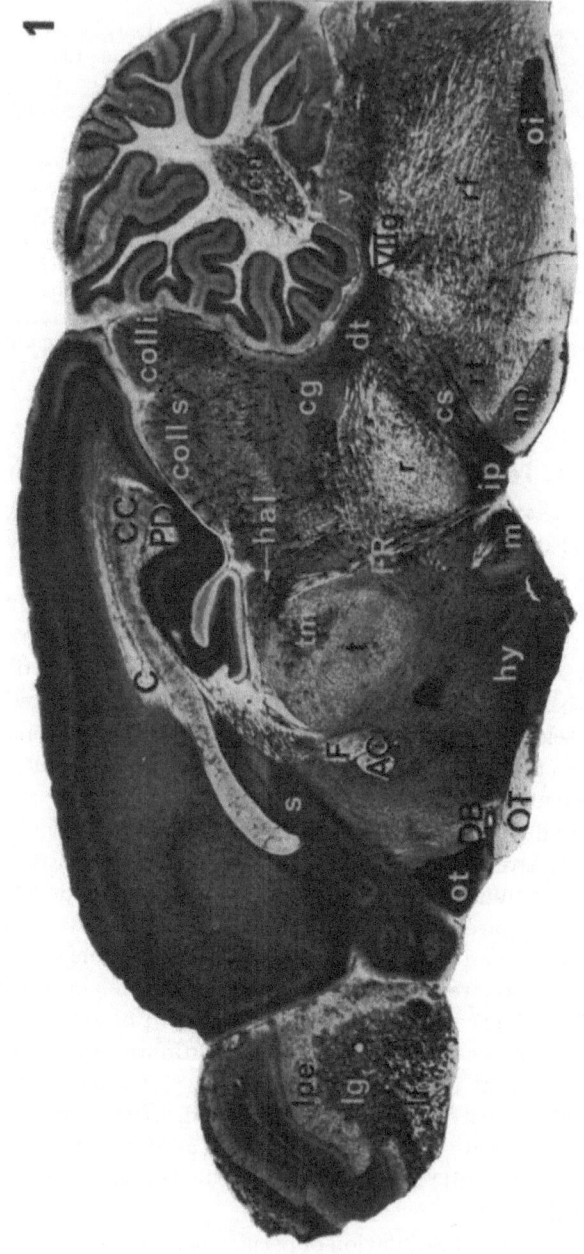

Fig. 1. Para-sagittal section ×6.7. This and all succeeding figures represent 40 micron thick cryostat sections, stained only with Timm's method unless otherwise stated. For abbreviations, see p. 7

strongly brown in incident or transmitted light. After 80 to 90 minutes, the colour is a dirty greyish brown as seen in incident light, but a clear red-brown in transmitted light.

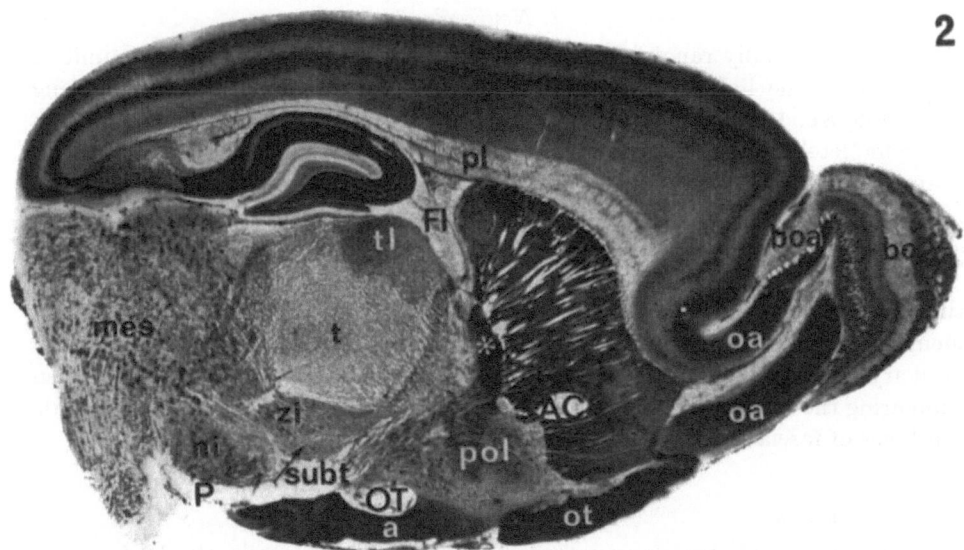

Fig. 2. Parasagittal section, × 6.7. Abbreviations, see p. 7. Asterisk on the bed nucleus of stria terminalis

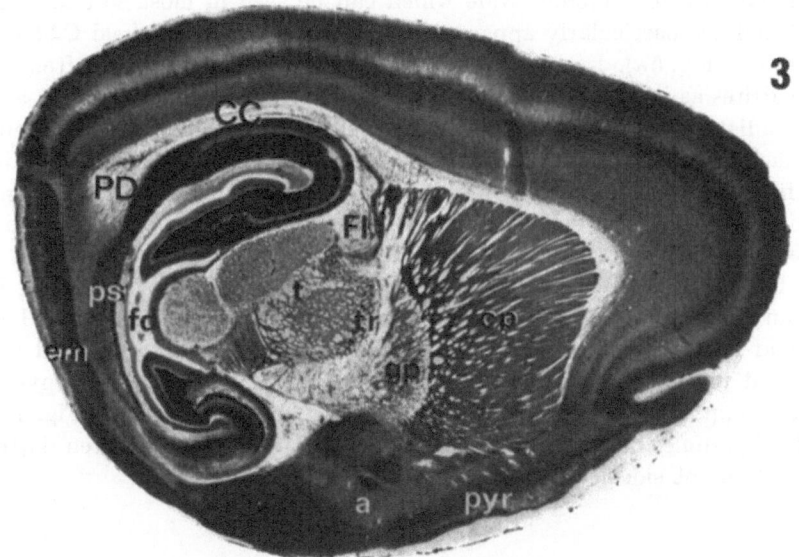

Fig. 3. Parasagittal section, × 6.7. Abbreviations, see p. 7

B. General Distribution of the Stain in Grey and White Matter

All major subdivisions of the rat central nervous system are stained. The telencephalon shows the strongest impregnation with the most striking regional differences but on prolonged development considerable differentiation appears also between individual nuclei and areas of the brain stem (Figs. 1–3). Troughout the brain the impregnation is located chiefly in grey matter.

1. Neuropil

Granules, usually ranging in size from about 2 microns down to the limit of resolution of the light microscope, account for the major part of the staining (Figs. 4–6, 8b, 16c, 18b). Only low power microscopy may give the impression of a completely diffuse background staining. Some areas contain larger particles than other areas as may be seen by comparing top and bottom of Fig. 5b. The hippocampal mossy fibre boutons (e.g., Fig. 2 of Haug, 1967) are far larger than any other stained particles.

Large grains within the neuropil usually but not invariably appear darker than smaller ones at a given submaximal degree of development. As already mentioned, grains in the neuropil are usually lighter than those associated with perikarya even when the neuropil grains are the larger (this is most marked when comparing the hippocampal mossy fibre boutons with, e.g., particles in the granule cell layer of fascia dentata).

a) Telencephalon

In the telencephalon the neuropil is more reactive than in the brain stem, spinal cord and cerebellum, due to a much higher concentration of strongly staining particles. These are evenly distributed (Figs. 4a–c, 5a, b, 6b, c) but tend to avoid stripes a few microns wide which can be seen in most cortical regions (Fig. 4c) and are particularly apparent in stratum radiatum of field CA1 of the hippocampus (Fig. 5a). In paraffin sections these unstained stripes often prove to be dendrites as is readily evident in parts of the neocortex (Fig. 4d, e) and in stratum radiatum of CA1 where thick pyramidal cell dendrites are arranged in parallel fashion (Fig. 5c, d). Other areas such as stratum radiatum of the hippocampal field CA3 (Fig. 5e) or the molecular layer of the fascia dentata (Fig. 6d) show thin, irregularly arranged, unstained stripes. Their appearance is consistent with the characteristic dendritic pattern of these areas.

Less frequently a distinct aggregation of stained granules occurs along both sides of an unstained stripe. This appearance is common in the basal and lateral amygdaloid nuclei of the cat (Fig. 7 of Hall, Haug and Ursin, 1969) and in the rat is found in the amygdala and some cortical areas including the pyriform cortex, the hippocampus (stratum oriens) and parts of the neocortex (Fig. 4a, b). The stained granules in the telencephalon are round or oblong and often flattened or indented on one side.

Fig. 4a—e. Character of the impregnation in neocortical neuropil. a) × 112. 10 micron cryostat section, counterstained with thionin. Note uniform distribution of impregnated particles throughout one layer (as opposed to patches in 8a). Note also barely resolvable dark lines, at arrows and elsewhere, and compare with b. b) × 1120. 40 micron cryostat section. Note the particulate nature of the impregnation as a whole and of two dark lines like those in a, appearing here as imperfect double rows of granules. c) × 1120. 3 micron cryostat section, weakly counterstained with thionin, showing one white stripe, possibly originating from one of the perikarya at the bottom. d) × 220; e) × 350. 15 micron paraffin section, counterstained with thionin. Note unstained dendrites in e, extending from layer V to layer I in d

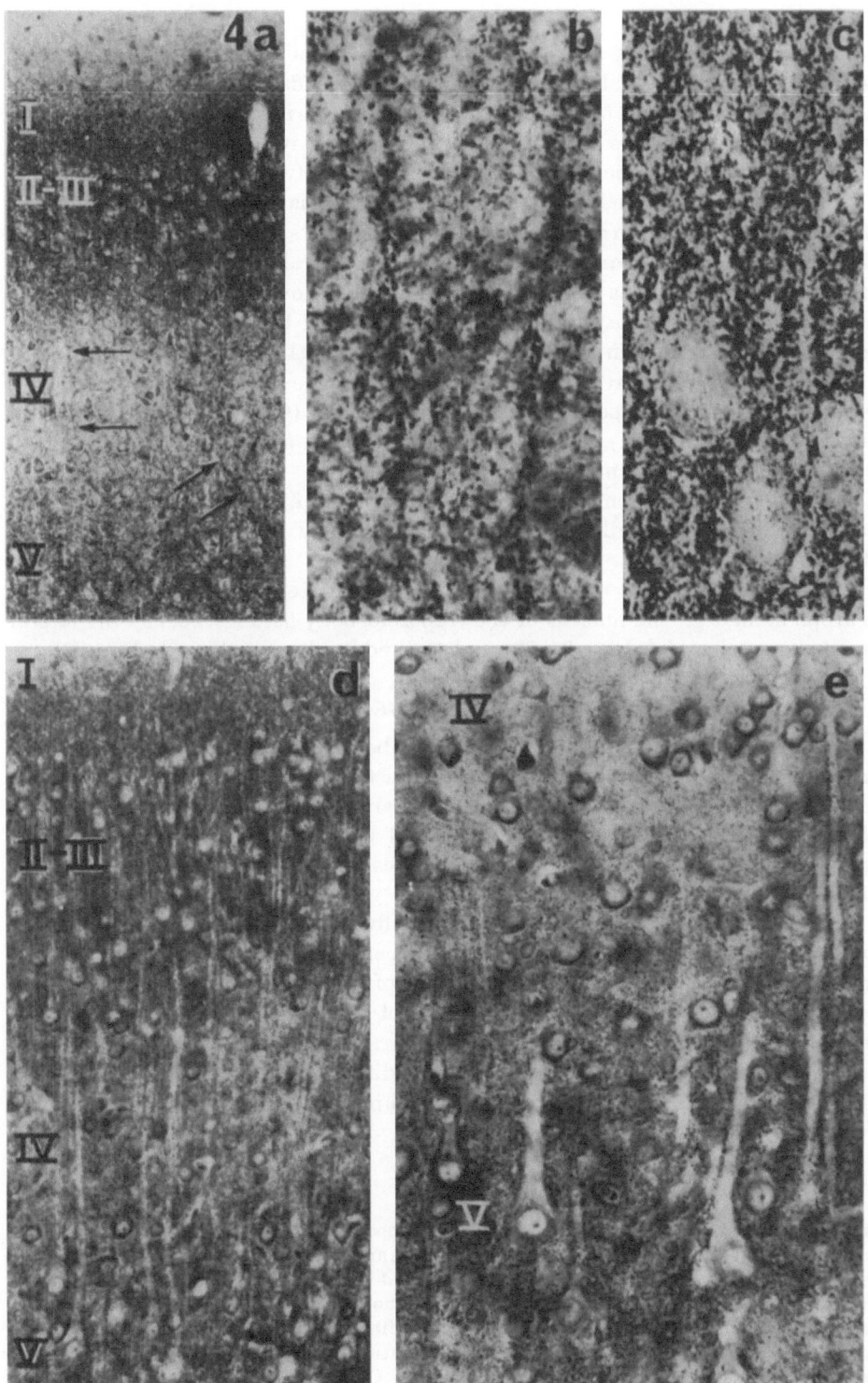

Fig. 4 a—e

b) Brain Stem

A significant part of the stainability of the brain stem neuropil appears to reside in glial processes, being confined to fine threads or strands (Fig. 16 d), as will be described below (5, p. 23). This results in perivascular patches of stain, which are typical of the mesencephalic tectum and reticular formation and of parts of the diencephalon, while occurring more rarely in the pons (Fig. 1).

In addition a uniform, fine grained, impregnation is found—most easily where the presumed glial impregnation is sparse, as in parts of the thalamus, most of the hypothalamus and part of the mesencephalic central grey (Figs. 1, 15 c, f, 16 a). High power micrographs of this staining are not shown here but the granules are comparable to those in the molecular layers of the fascia dentata or the cerebellum (p. 43), and in some regions even less reactive.

The neuropil of many circumscribed nuclei in the brain stem, i.e., the nigra (ni, Fig. 16 a), the interpeduncular nucleus (ip, Fig. 16 a), the dorsal tegmental nucleus (dt, Figs. 18 a, 31), and of the cerebellar nuclei (cn, Figs. 18 a, 34–37) show a particularly strong granular staining.

In the pontine and medullary reticular formation scattered granules occur between the fibre bundles. They are often clearly located within dendrites (Fig. 17 b).

It is interesting that certain areas of the brain stem are virtually devoid of neuropil stain, e.g., the nucleus of the trapezoid body (ct, Figs. 28, 29), the lateral vestibular nucleus (vl, Figs. 31–33) and the red nucleus (r, Figs. 1, 16 a, 28).

2. Neuronal Perikarya

Staining of neuronal perikarya was described by Timm (1958 a, 1961), Brun and Brunk (1970) and others. It usually consists of distinct particles ranging up to 2 microns in diameter. The size, intracellular distribution and packing density of the stained particles differ regionally and between types of neurons within any one region. A few of these characteristics will be mentioned when the individual regions are described.

In the telencephalon, the granules are usually confined to the somata; in many lower centres they are also present quite far peripherally in dendrites (Fig. 17 b). In a few instances a pericellular localization of the stained granules may not be definitively excluded, e.g., in the cell layers of the fascia dentata (gran, Fig. 6 a) and particularly in hippocampal field CA1 (arrows, Fig. 5 a).

Some neuronal somata have an additional diffuse background staining (faintly visible in the photomicrograph of Fig. 17 b). Finally some somata, such as those

Fig. 5 a—e. Details of the impregnation in the hippocampus. a) × 450. Field CA1. Note granules (arrows) in apical position on or within pyramidal cells (pyr) and light striation of neuropil in stratum radiatum (rad). b) × 1120. Field CA1. Note that impregnated granules located in the deepest part of stratum lacunosum moleculare (lac) are larger than those in radiatum (rad). c) × 220; d) × 950. 15 micron paraffin sections. Unstained dendrites of CA1 pyramids (d) extending throughout the depth of stratum radiatum (c). e) × 1440. 15 micron paraffin section, counterstained with thionin. From CA3 close to fascia dentata ("CA3c") in stratum radiatum at a level immediately below the border with lacunosum moleculare. Lighter stripes may represent unstained dendrites

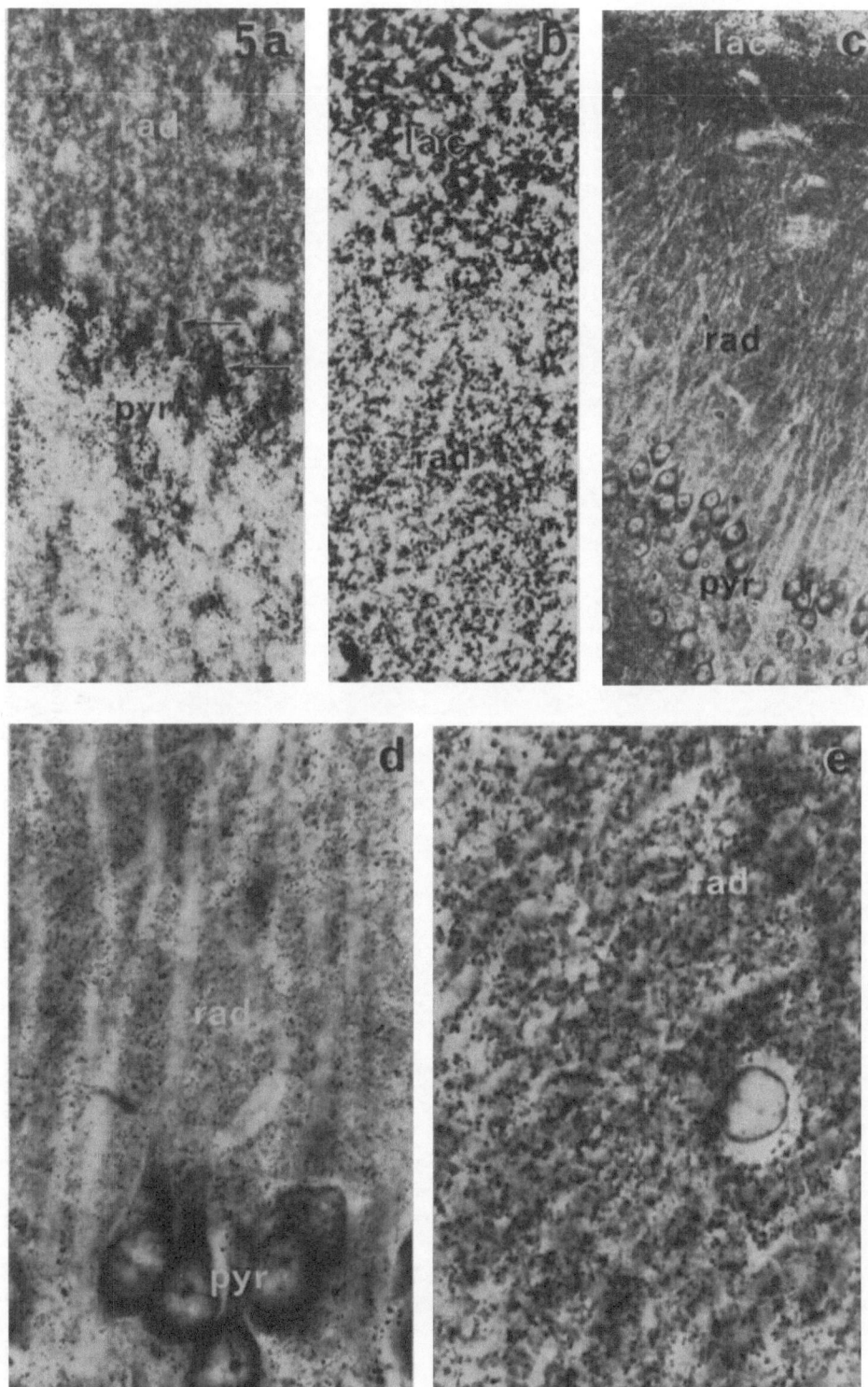

Fig. 5a—e

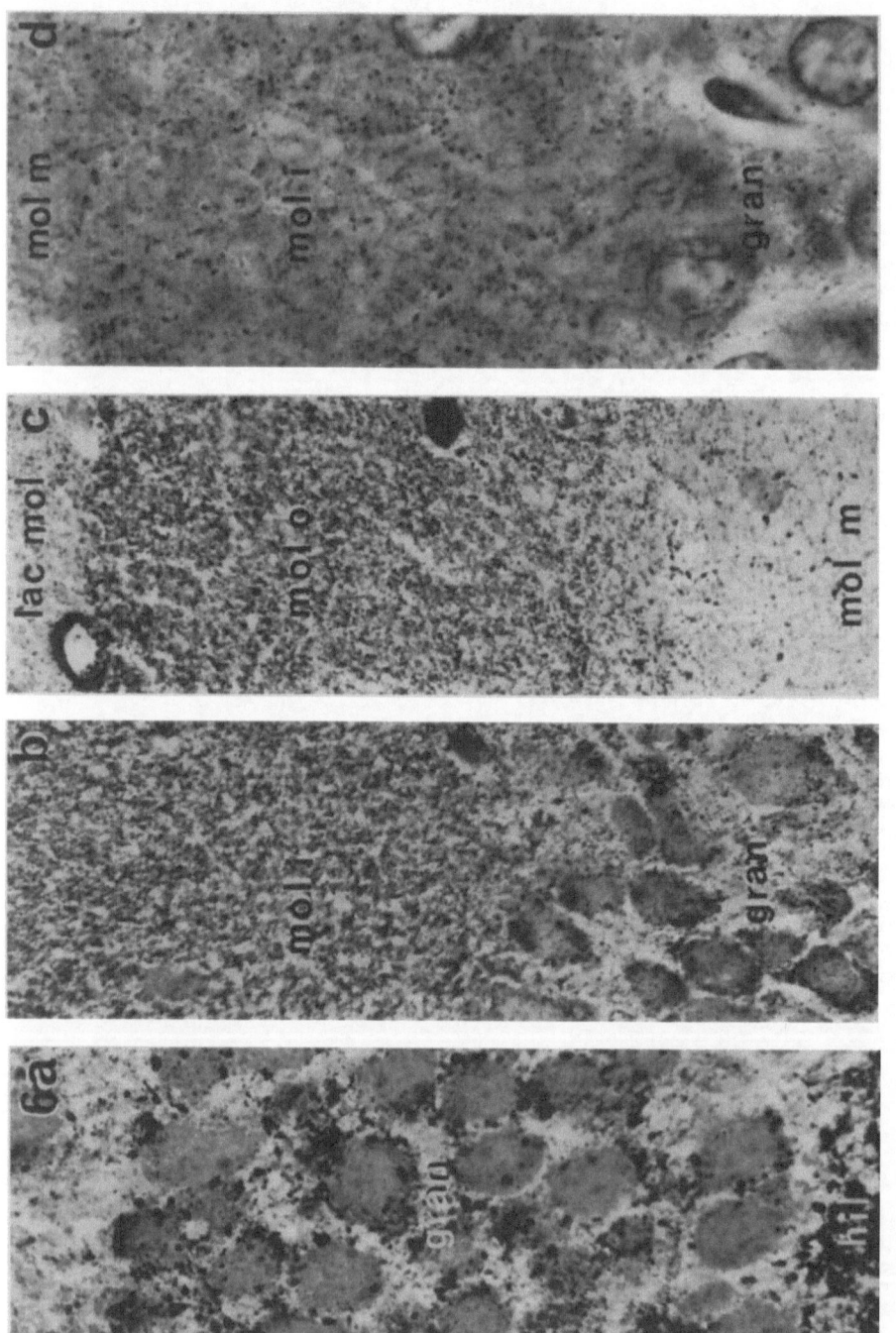

Fig. 6a—d. Details of the impregnation in fascia dentata. a) × 1120. 5 micron cryostat section, counterstained with thionin. Nuclei in the granule cell layer (*gran*) surrounded by large black granules. At the bottom, mossy fibre boutons in the hilus (*hil*). b) × 1120. 3 micron cryostat section, counterstained with thionin. Inner zone of molecular layer (*mol i*). Granule cell layer (*gran*) at the bottom. c) × 1120. 3 micron cryostat section, counterstained with thionin. Part of middle zone (*mol m*) together with outer zone (*mol o*) of molecular layer. At top, part of adjacent lacunosum moleculare (*lac mol*) of CA1. d) × 1440. 15 micron paraffin section, counterstained with thionin. Abbreviations as in a—c. The light striation best discernible in d, could well result from a lack of staining of larger dendrites

in the anterior olfactory nucleus (Fig. 12a) or layer IV of area entorhinalis, are completely nonreactive in the present material.

3. Neuroglia and Vessels

a) Glial Cells

The classification of glial cells constitutes a particular field of study outside the scope of the present article. It is nevertheless desirable to render here a first description of impregnation which is believed to reveal glial perikarya and processes. The following arbitrary categories (paragraphs *1* to *6*) are not intended to be rigidly interpreted in terms of established glial cell types. Attempts at an interpretation are presented below (p. 56).

1. Cells with fusiform to round perikarya, black as if impregnated by a Golgi method, and with a few well stained, irregular processes (Fig. 7a).

The perikarya are of variable size, roughly 5×15 microns (15 microns if round). A pale nucleus is apparent in some cells. The processes show considerable variation in regard to thickness, degree of branching and general disposition, but are always few, irregular, branch at wide angles and keep within some 50 microns of their perikarya. The whole cell or its processes occasionally adhere to the wall of medium sized vessels.

These cells are scattered singly or—occasionally—in small groups throughout grey and white matter. They are rare except in the corpus callosum, the dorsal psalterium (Fig. 7b), the external capsule (Fig. 7a) and the central grey matter (obliterated ventricle) of the olfactory bulb (where the processes are less well developed, Fig. 7c). Forms transitional between these and those described in *2* are also seen.

2. Cells with oval to round perikarya and thin processes stained only at their departure from the perikaryon (Fig. 8e).

The pale, round nuclei often leave only a narrow rim of black cytoplasm (black arrows, Fig. 8e), while other perikarya appear black throughout (white arrows, Fig. 8e). Some of these perikarya lie free in the neuropil or at the periphery of fibre bundles, but most of them are located in the vicinity of vessels or adhere to vessels, singly or in rows (arrows, Figs. 8c, 16d).

These cells are common in both white and grey matter. There are striking regional differences in their number, however. Thus, grey matter in the forebrain is virtually devoid of such cells—whether free in the neuropil or accompanying vessels—while some parts of the brain stem abound with them, especially the pallidum (Figs. 8a, c), the interpeduncular nucleus (Figs. 16a, c), the tegmentum dorsal to the latter (Figs. 1, 8d, e), and the mesencephalic tectum and tegmentum as a whole. In general, their number seems to correlate with the presence and intensity of the perivascular patches to be described (*5*, p. 23).

Various fibre tracts also differ with regard to the number of such cells.

3. Cells—with several smooth, straight processes—which even after strong development are faintly stained except for a few black particles (Fig. 9a, b).

The processes branch at acute angles and extend for 100 microns or more avay from the parent perikarya. They often connect with the walls of vessels or

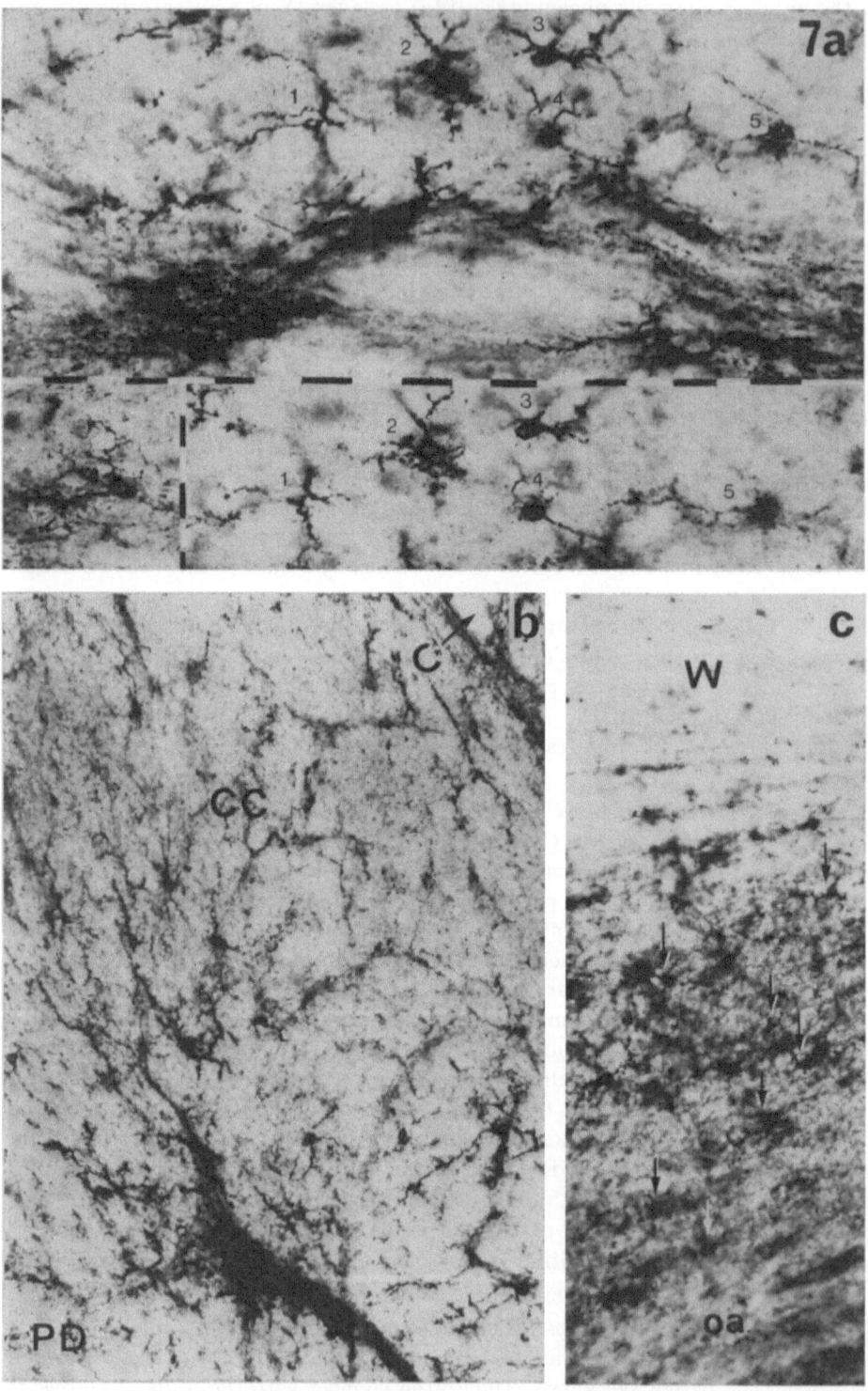

Fig. 7 a—c

with the pia (Fig. 9b). Glial cells of this type predominate in most fibre tracts. Tangles formed by processes arising from several perikarya then appear as diffuse patches along vessels. However, certain fibre tracts, particularly the corpus callosum, show few stained cells of this type.

4. *Aggregates of round, fairly large, black, granules* are found everywhere in white matter with short periods of development (arrow, Fig. 10a). Individual granules vary from less than 1 micron up to 2 micron diameter. Counterstaining with thionine reveals their close relation to cells that often form part of a row of oligoglial cells, particularly so in the corpus callosum. Only a few of the cells in these rows are associated with Timm stained granules, however.

On stronger development, it becomes apparent that some of these granules belong to perikarya or proximal processes of cells described under 3, while others probably belong to cells similar to those described under 2 or 1 but requiring particularly strong development to be entirely visualized.

Similar aggregates of granules are numerous in some cortical areas or laminae such as stratum lacunosum moleculare (arrow, Fig. 10b) and stratum radiatum (arrow, Fig. 10c) of CA1, but here their parent cells are not revealed even by prolonged development.

5. *Diffuse patches of stain surrounding medium sized vessels* (asterisk, Fig. 8a, Figs. 8c, 15b, 16a, d) are found in parts of the diencephalon (including the pallidum) and in the mesencephalon (Figs. 1, 16a, 29). Being some tens of microns wide they usually surround vessels of 5 to 30 microns diameter. They consist of distinct dark granules and more faintly stainable strands or threads as seen at high magnifications (arrowheads, Figs. 8c, 16d). Dark cells resembling those described above under 2 or (more rarely) 1 contribute to the stain in these patches.

Many parts of the brain stem, some of which contain a significant amount of evenly distributed granular stain, are virtually devoid of such perivascular patches, e.g., large parts of the hypothalamus (Figs. 15c, d, f), the reticular tegmental nucleus (Fig. 17c), and—to a variable extent—the periaqueductal grey (*cg*, Figs. 16a, 29, 30; compare Figs. 40a, c).

6. To complete the present list it should be mentioned that in some series, particularly in the pallidum, thicker and darker threads and granules are also found within fibre bundles being oriented along the fibres (not illustrated). The appearance is not that of a conventional axon or myelin stain but is consistent with the staining of glial processes.

Fig. 7a—c. Impregnation of glial cells (*1*, p. 21). a) × 450. From the external capsule. Cells 1—5 shown also below broken line in a slightly different focus. b) × 220. From the splenium of corpus callosum with adjacent cingulum and dorsal psalterium. Throughout the field numerous cells similar to those shown in a. c) × 220. From the obliterated olfactory ventricle. A few perikarya are well focused in the thick section and some of these are indicated by arrows. The dark background results mainly from numerous stained cells of similar appearance being out of focus. *W* central white matter of olfactory bulb, *oa* inner layer of anterior olfactory nucleus

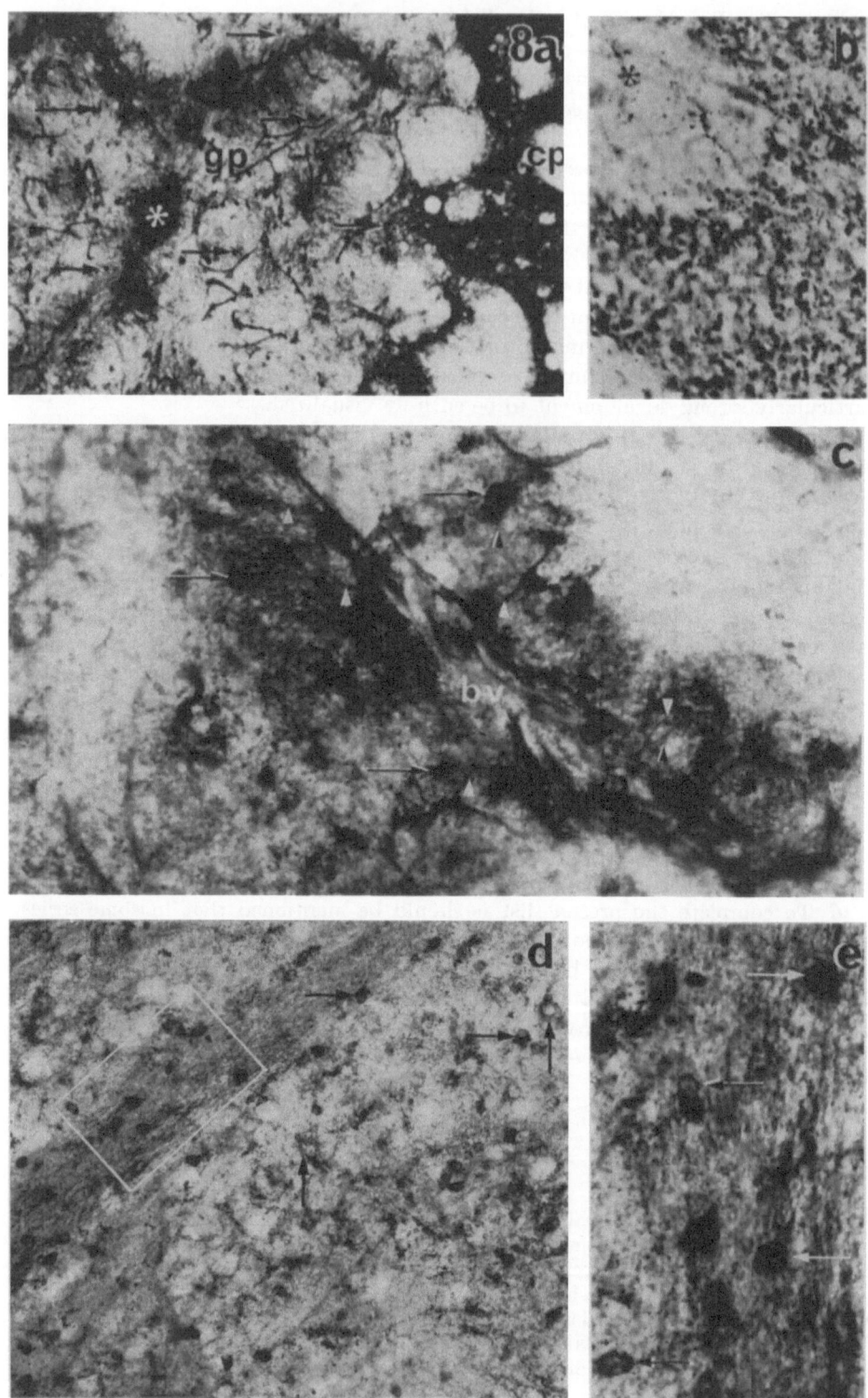

Fig. 8a—e

b) Ependyma and Choroid Plexus

The staining of the choroid plexus (*pl*, Fig. 11) and the ependyma (Fig. 15 d) often ranges from heavy to none at all within one and the same series (Figs. 21 to 23, 26–27, 34–37). Parts of the ventricles or subarachnoid space adjacent to the ependyma or choroid plexus are often diffusely impregnated (Fig. 18 b). In one brain, basal extensions of ependymal cells (tanycyte processes, Horstmann, 1954; Leonhardt, 1966; and others) were stained along a restricted sector of the lateral wall of the third ventricle. These processes were smooth and slender and coursed for long distances (Fig. 15 d), often terminating on a vessel. Ten other brains examined did not show this particular phenomenon. More frequently, similar, thicker processes were found in the ventral wall of the infundibular recess. (Basal ependymal processes occur more generally than would appear from the few stained in Fig. 15 d; see Bleier, 1971.)

c) Vessels

Throughout the central nervous system vessels with diameters up to 30 microns show a staining which appears confined to a thin layer within, or possibly on the outside of their walls (Figs. 8 c, 9 a, b, 16 d, 17). This stain consists of granules, roughly 1 micron and less in diameter, and distinct "strings" of similar thickness, which run longitudinally, branching every now and then. A few of the strings prove to be processes of perivascular glial cells as described above (Figs. 8 c, 9 b). As already mentioned, sulphide silver stainable glia (*3*, or *2*, and *5*) surround the vessels in some, but not all parts of the brain.

4. Axons and Myelin

No part of the central nervous system shows any indication of staining of single axons or fibre bundles resembling that seen with Golgi methods, reduced

Fig. 8 a—e. Impregnation of glial cells (*2*, p. 21 and *5*, p. 23). a) × 112. Globus pallidus (*gp*). Small black perikarya scattered between the fibre bundles and along vessels (asterisk) where in the photomicrograph they are obscured by dense filamentous impregnation shown at higher magnification in c. Compare the patchy character of the impregnation in globus pallidus with the uniform, profuse, granular staining of the neuropil in adjacent striatum (*cp*, further enlarged in b. b) × 1120. 5 micron cryostat section. From the striatum. Note uniform scattering of distinct particles. c) × 440. Globus pallidus. Tangentially sectioned vessel (*bv*). Thread-like character of the perivascular impregnation may be discerned (arrow heads). Note small dark cells (arrows and elsewhere) with poorly stained processes. d) × 220. Sagittal section. Nucleus centralis superior (cp. survey picture of Fig. 1) contains small round glial perikarya (horizontal arrows) and dorsobasally oriented stained "threads" (further enlarged in e). Vertical arrows indicate neurons with granular staining in perikarya and dendrites. e) × 570. Frame in d further enlarged. Black and white arrows on glial perikarya where the pale nucleus is visible. White arrows on perikarya where the nucleus is obscured. The dorsobasally oriented threads probably represent processes of the small round glial perikarya

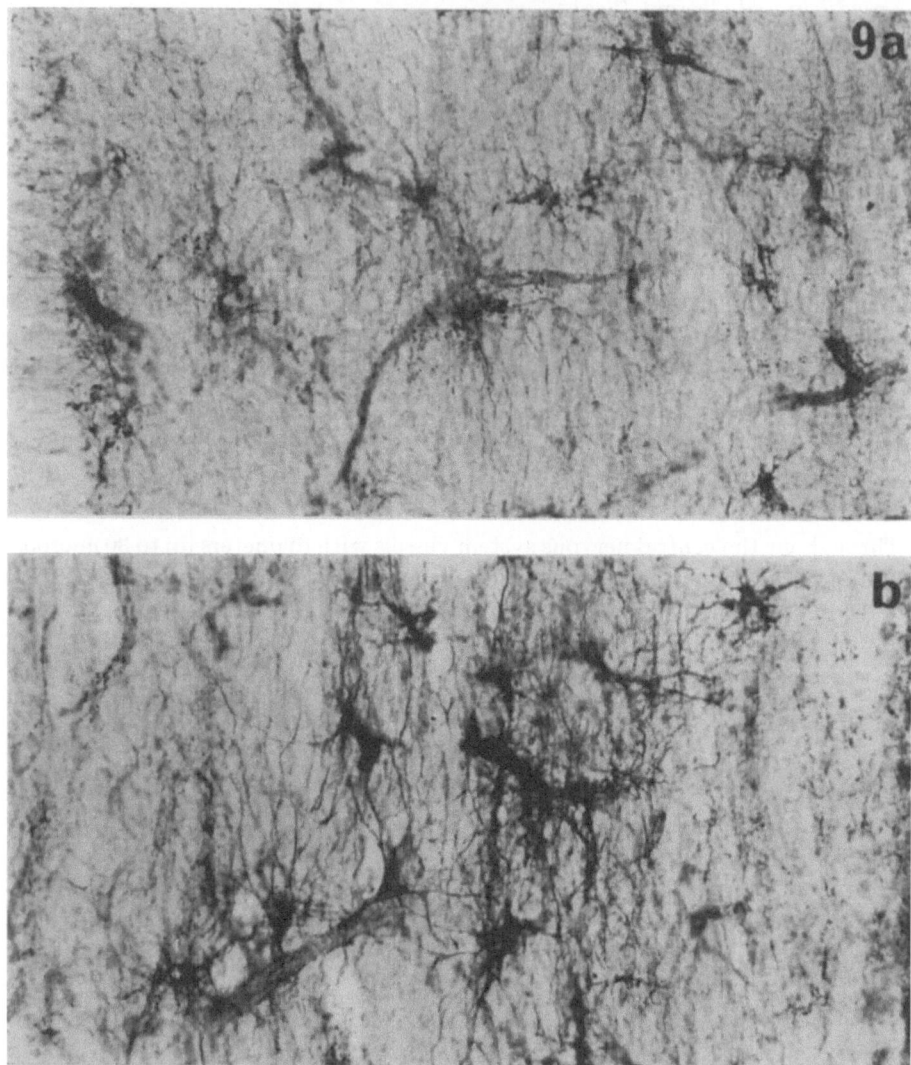

Fig. 9a and b. × 350. Impregnation of glial cells (*3*, p. 21). a) and b) are both from tractus spinalis of the trigeminal nerve within the same uniformly stained series, yet the cells shown in a are less completely stained than in b. Note frequent vascular insertions of processes and occasional perivascular position of perikarya

silver methods or myelin stains. White matter in general is weakly reactive, its staining being apparently confined mainly to glia as described above. After strong development (70 to 90 minutes), some fibre tracts show a weak stain confined to vessels and to glial perikarya and processes (*CI*, Fig. 11a; *PD*, *C*, Fig. 11b), some show a more profuse patchy staining (*ST*, Fig. 11a) and some (*CC*, Fig. 11b) show a diffuse stain, the localization of which cannot be deduced.

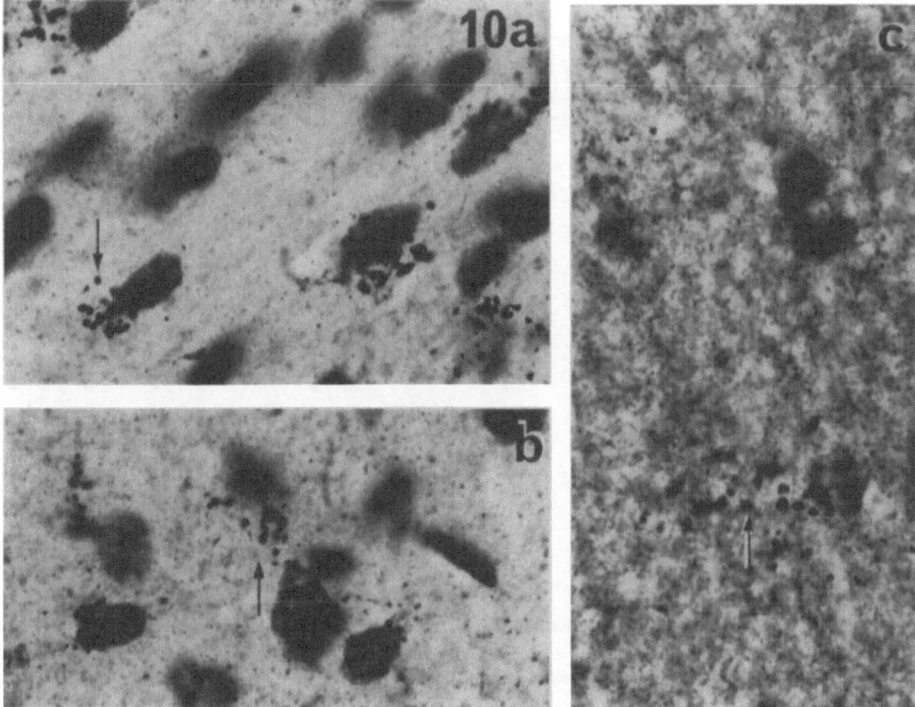

Fig. 10a—c. × 1120. Glial impregnation (4, p. 23). Sections counterstained with thionin to visualize the nuclei. a) From the corpus callosum. b) From stratum lacunosum moleculare of hippocampal field CA1. c) From stratum radiatum of field CA1. Note difference in size and apparent density between perinuclear (glial) and neuropil granules

C. Regional Staining Patterns

1. Telencephalon

Neuropil (p. 16) and neuronal perikarya (p. 18) contain most of the stain. It is especially noteworthy that the small round glial cells (2, p. 21) and the perivascular patches, so abundant in parts of the brain stem, are absent from grey matter in the forebrain, except the olfactory bulb.

In the *olfactory bulb* (Fig. 12) the fibrillary layer contains densely stained patches which are irregularly distributed and show diffuse limits (Fig. 12a). At higher magnification this stain is resolved into grains and strands surrounding vessels and encroaching on the fibre bundles (asterisks, Fig. 12b). Furthermore, numerous glial perikarya are seen (but not illustrated here). The majority of these fit the description in paragraph 2, p. 21. Quite a few have somewhat better developed processes, however, and occasional cells correspond entirely to those described in paragraph 1, p. 21.

The stain in the fibrillary layer extends into the glomerular layer where it partially covers the superficial aspects of the glomeruli (*gl*, Fig. 12b). The glomer-

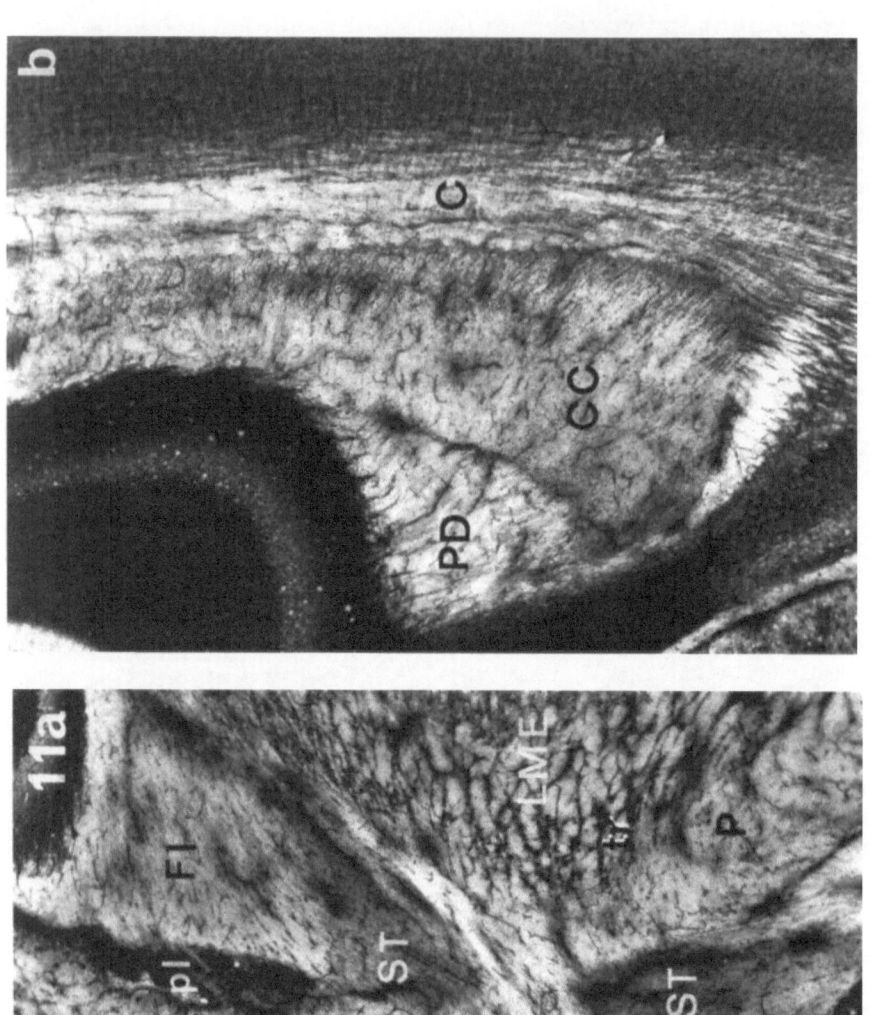

Fig. 11 a and b. × 35. Impregnation of vessels and of diffuse perivascular patches in compact white matter. Slight differences in the character and amount of impregnation between some of the large fibre tracts. a) The internal capsule, the cerebral peduncle and the fornix are pale except for perivascular patches of impregnation. By contrast a more pronounced, uniform, staining is seen in the stria terminalis. b) Corpus callosum shows an evenly distributed "background" impregnation in addition to perivascular patches. Dorsal psalterium a little paler than the corpus callosum. Cingulum and particularly the fibre bundles behind the splenium practically devoid of impregnation

uli themselves contain finer grains. Their strength of staining varies from series to series as does the sharpness of their outline (Fig. 12 b strikes about an average in both respects). Scattered dark granules are associated with the periglomerular cells (barely visible in Fig. 12 b).

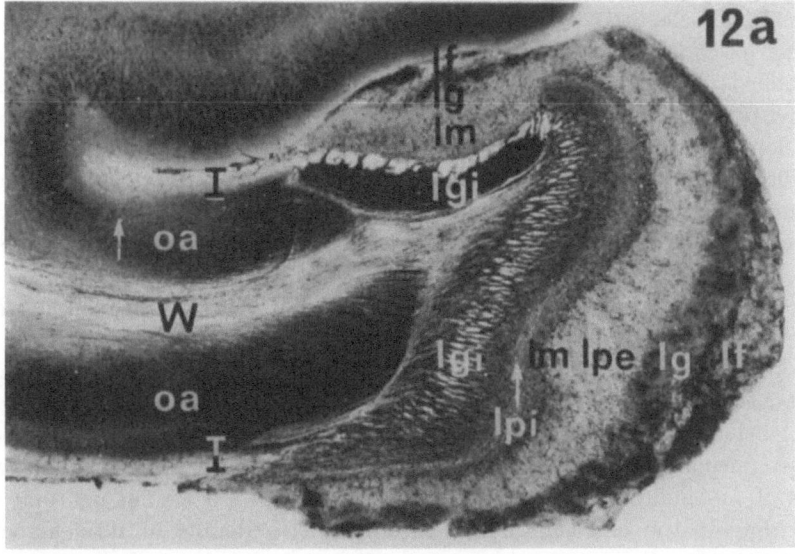

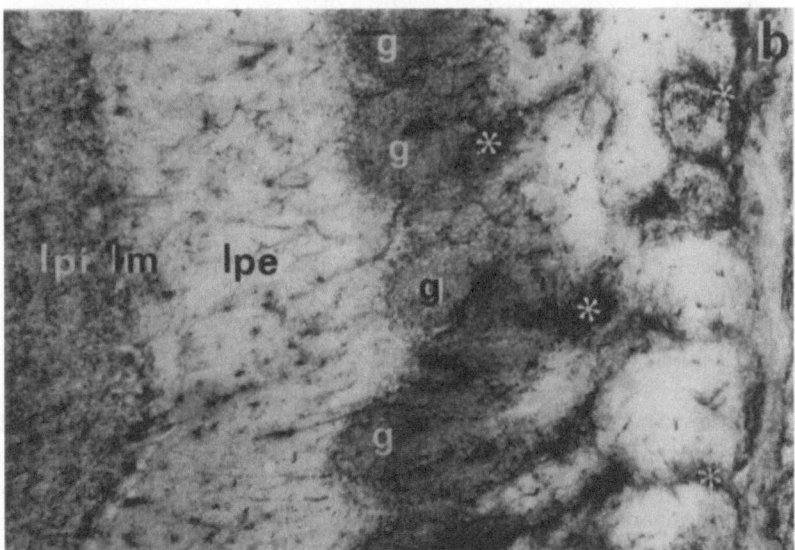

Fig. 12. a) × 18.6; b) × 88. Abbreviations not entered in list on p. 7: *g* glomeruli, *lgi* lamina granularis interna, *lm* lamina cellularum mitralium, *lpi* lamina plexiformis interna. Asterisk in b indicates patches of dense granular and filamentous staining often surrounding vessels. Although present in the field, numerous small black glial cells (see text *1* and *2*, p. 21) are not visible at this low magnification

    The neuropil of the external plexiform layer is light brown but paler than the glomeruli (*lpe*, Fig. 12b). A slight local increase of the staining density often occurs in the proximity of capillaries. Many perikarya of this zone show a distinct granular staining.

The mitral cells are covered or filled with large black granules (*lm*, Fig. 12b). The inner plexiform layer (*lpi*) is somewhat paler than the internal granular layer (*lgi*) which is dark and contains a brown, finely granular stain in the neuropil (avoiding fibre bundles) and larger black grains associated with the granule cells. In the depth of the internal granular layer several glial cells similar to those in the fibillary layer are present, which is exceptional in telencephalic grey matter. The central white matter is virtually unstained except for the glial cells which are especially numerous in the periventricular layer (arrows, Fig. 7c; *1*, p. 21).

The *accessory olfactory bulb* (Fig. 12a) will be described with reference to the laminae recognized by Lohman in the guinea pig (1963), since Nissl stained sections of the present material agree well with that description.

The fibrillary layer is lightly stained and the glomerular layer even more so. The external and internal plexiform layers and the interposed mitral layer show a homogeneous staining of the neuropil of low to medium density. Additional larger granules are associated with the mitral cells. Finally, below the unstained bundles of myelinated fibres the granular layer shows a strong neuropil stain (darker than in the olfactory bulb, see Fig. 12a) and dots of stain associated with the granule cells.

All parts of the *anterior olfactory nucleus* (Fig. 12a) show a profuse neuropil stain, except the lateral olfactory tract and a further outer part of the zonal layer which are unstained. The somata are constantly unstained, even when the perikarya of most other cortical regions are successfully impregnated.

The *olfactory tubercle* (*ot*, Figs. 1, 2, 19, 20) stains strongly throughout all layers except in an outer zone of layer I. The stain is located both to neuropil and somata. When the superficial curved layer of densely packed somata is traced in Nissl sections, a variation in size and packing density of the cells is apparent. Short stretches of smaller and more tightly packed cells often form sharp, superficially directed, convex bends of the cell layer. These segments of the layer are particularly strongly stained in the Timm sections (not illustrated). Furthermore, neuropil and cells in the islands of Calleja, deep to the superficial cell layer, stain particularly intensely as does the large island located medial to the nucleus accumbens (Fig. 19). Indeed, the reactivity of the cellular parts of these islands is comparable to that of the hippocampal mossy fibre layer. The small adjacent areas devoid of perikarya have a strong red tinge found nowhere else in the brain. At high magnifications this precipitate is seen to be very finely granular.

The *substriatal grey*, the *substantia innominata*, and the *lateral preoptic region* are poorly defined and to a large extent overlapping in the rat (see Price and Powell, 1970). For the purpose of a first description of the sulphide silver pattern, these terms will in the present report be used interchangeably to indicate the area (Figs. 19–21) dorsal and posterior to the posterior part of the olfactory tubercle. It is limited by the striatum dorsally, and merges with the globus pallidus posterodorsally (*gp*, Fig. 21), with the lateral hypothalamic region posteriorly (*hl*, Fig. 22), and with the anterior amygdaloid area (*aaa*, Fig. 21) posterolaterally at the level of the nucleus of the olfactory tract. In the part of this territory which contains the nucleus of the horizontal limb of the diagonal band (Price and Powell, 1970), the neuropil is virtually nonreactive (asterisks in Figs. 20 to 21), just as in the nucleus of the vertical limb (*DB*, Figs. 19–20). The remaining parts of the area have the same patchy impregnation as the globus pallidus and the anterior part of the lateral hypothalamic area. The whole territory is conspicuously paler than, and sharply delimited from, the olfactory tubercle and the striatum (Figs. 19–21) and differs from the anterior amygdaloid area which stains more homogeneously (*aaa*, Fig. 21). It sends an extension rostrally between the olfactory tubercle and the striatum-accumbens (Figs. 2, 19). At these rostral levels, ventral extensions of the striatum (vertical arrow, Fig. 19) divide the pale area into partially separate fields which correspond in general disposition to fascicles of the medial forebrain bundle (as represented by König and Klippel, 1963).

The *septal area* (Figs. 19–21; *s*, Figs. 1, 40 c) reveals a varied staining pattern, particularly in the neuropil; diffuse gradients are more common than sharp limits. The anterior continuation of the hippocampus is clearly visible having an unstained "granular layer" and a molecular layer subdivided into a superficial pale and deeper dark part (not illustrated here; see Haug, 1973). The bed nucleus of stria terminalis is dark (asterisk, Fig. 2; *st*, Fig. 21), that of the anterior commissure being somewhat paler. The two structures grade into each other and into the adjacent, lighter, septal and hypothalamic areas. The medial septal nucleus or a medial part of it is very pale (*sm*, Fig. 19) and thus inseparable from the nucleus of the diagonal band (*DB* and asterisks, Figs. 19–21), while the lateral nucleus is darker. Within the latter (*sl*, Figs. 19–21; see also Fig. 40 c), several gradients of staining are visible in the neuropil. Neuronal perikarya also show some regional differences in staining.

The *amygdaloid nuclei* (Figs. 21–25) show a Timm-pattern resembling that seen in the cat (Hall, Haug, and Ursin, 1969). The cortical, basal and parts of the lateral and central nuclei (Brodal, 1947) are strongly stained. Parts of the central, lateral and medial nuclei are more weakly stained. A sharply delimited superficial zone in the cortical and medial nuclei is wholly unstained.

In the *caudate-putamen* (Figs. 19–24) perikarya are stained but the neuropil contributes most of the density. Its stained granules are evenly distributed (Fig. 8 b), sharply avoiding the fibre bundles. A slightly increased staining is apparent along part of the medial border (Figs. 2, 3, 19–24). The striatum is delimited sharply from the pallidum and substriatal grey (Figs. 2, 3, 19–23) but more vaguely from the amygdala (*a*, Figs. 3, 22–24).

The *nucleus accumbens septi* (Figs. 19–20) is less reactive than the rest of the striatum, from which it is indistinctly delimited. Within the neuropil of the accumbens and adjoining parts of the caudate-putamen there are moderate local variations in staining density (Figs. 2, 19–20) which seem to bear some relation to faint cytoarchitectonic variations. As in Nissl sections the septal border is distinct (Figs. 19–20).

In the *cerebral cortex* both neuropil and perikarya are well stained (Figs. 12 a, 14, 19). The neuropil makes the most substantial contribution to the total staining of the cortex if the sections are not too weakly stained (see section III-A). Laminar and interareal differences are evident with respect to neuropil as well as perikarya. Gradual transitions rather than sharp limits are the rule. However, the cingulate cortex (its superficial layers Fig. 27), the pyriform cortex (Fig. 3) and particularly the hippocampal formation (Fig. 14) display several sharp interlaminar and interareal limits.

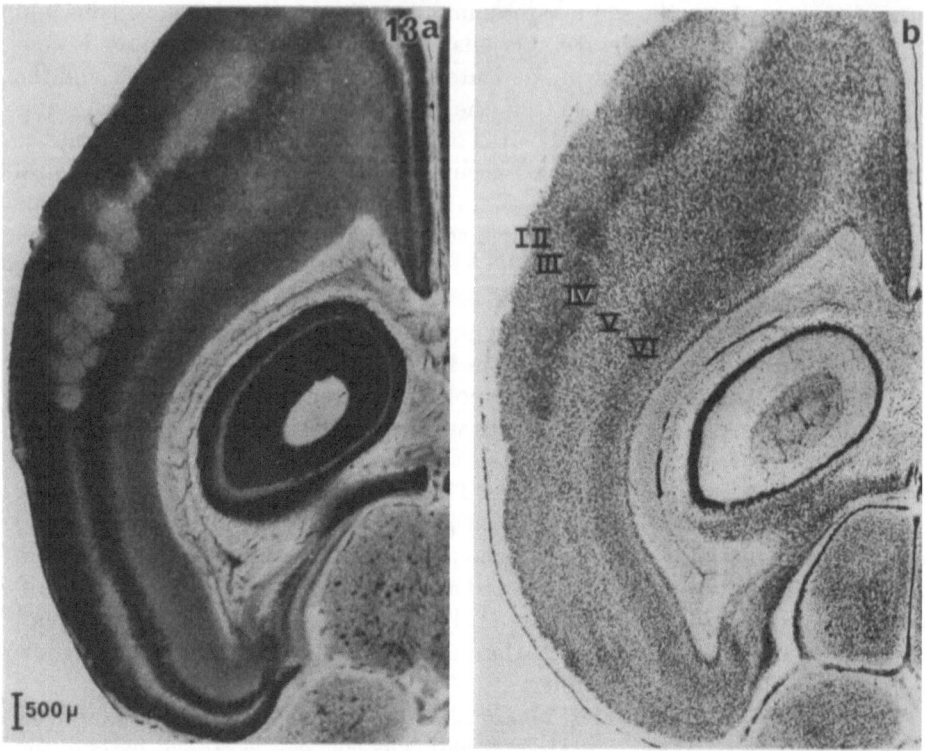

Fig. 13a and b. × 8.7. a) Timm-stained. b) Thionin-stained. *I–VI* Cortical layers. The outer dark zone in the Timm-pattern corresponds roughly to an inner part of layer I together with layers II and III. The inner dark zone in the Timm pattern is at least partly coexistant with layer V. In somatosensory cortex, extensions of stained neuropil from layer V into IV, should be noted. They delimit paler fields corresponding roughly to the rounded cell rich fields in the thionin section (see text p. 32)

It is not intended here to give a detailed analysis of the staining pattern of individual areas; only a few conspicuous features will be mentioned.

Within the *neocortex* the neuropil is heavily stained in two zones extending continuously through all areas (Figs. 1–3, 13, 14, 19, 20, 27). The outer dark zone (see Fig. 13a, b) covers the deeper and major part of layer I together with layers II and III. The inner dark zone covers part or all of layer V. A pale zone superficially in layer I varies in depth and distinctness between different regions. Another pale zone is approximately congruent with layer IV.

In a region roughly corresponding to the somatosensory area the pale layer IV has a distinct and peculiarly serrated deep border. Sagittal or horizontal sections, passing obliquely through this area, reveal several rounded pale fields, separated by slightly darker extensions from layer V (Fig. 13a, b). These fields undoubtedly reflect the barrels of layer IV (Woolsey and van der Loos, 1970; Welker, 1971), although corresponding round fields seen in the adjacent thionine stained sections (Fig. 13b) lack central hollows and appear slightly larger than

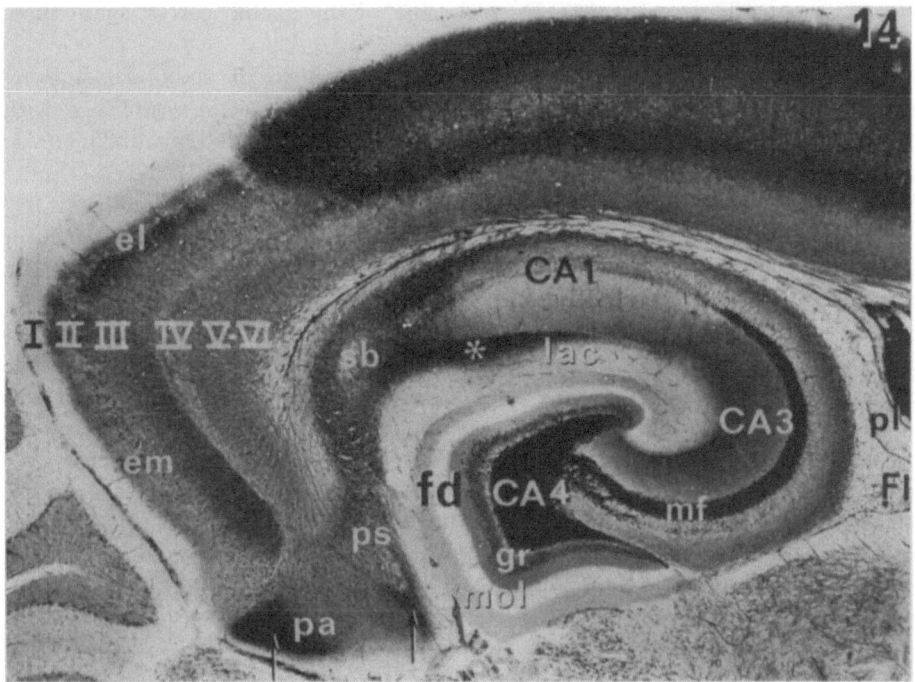

Fig. 14. × 26. Hippocampal region, horizontal section. Abbreviations not entered in list p. 7: *I–VI* entorhinal layers, *CA1–CA4* hippocampal fields, *gr* granule cell layer of fascia dentata, *lac* stratum lacunosum moleculare of the hippocampus, *mol* molecular layer of fascia dentata, *mf* mossy fibre layer of CA3, *pa* the parasubiculum, *sb* the subiculum. Asterisk indicates darkly stained wedge extending from inner zone of subiculum into deepest part of stratum lacunosum of CA1. For further description (see text p. 34)

individual barrels as previously described (respective diameters are 250–500 microns and 150–400 microns).

In the vicinity of the rhinal fissure where layer IV dwindles (Krieg, 1946), the middle pale zone also becomes narrower so that eventually the outer and inner dark zones fuse in the areas adjoining the pyriform and entorhinal cortices. The density of the dark zones is increased somewhat in these areas (Figs. 14, 19–20).

Layer VI appears homogeneous and fairly weakly stained. At the deep border of layer V there is often a diffusely delimited narrow zone, slightly paler than layer VI (Figs. 3, 19, 20). The border between grey and white matter is always sharp.

The above description concerns only the staining of neuropil. Perikarya are stained in all layers (Figs. 12a, 19). Larger pyramidal cells of layer III, and particularly of layer V, stain particularly strongly (see also Brun and Brunk, 1970).

The *cingulate cortex* (Domesick, 1969). The retrosplenial areas (areas 29b and c of Krieg, 1946; retrosplenial and posterior cingular areas of Rose and Woolsey, 1948) are sharply delimited and reveal a conspicuous lamination of the stain in

neuropil and perikarya (Fig. 27). Rostral parts of the medial cortex again show
a more diffuse layering (Fig. 19).

The *hippocampal formation* (Figs. 1–3, 14) displays an elaborate staining
pattern intimately related to the laminar and areal subdivision established with
conventional histological methods (Cajal, 1911; Lorente de Nó, 1933, 1934;
Blackstad, 1956; and others).

In the fascia dentata the molecular layer is sharply trilaminar (*mol*, Fig. 14),
with a virtually unstained middle zone (*mol m*, Fig. 6c), a lightly stained outer
zone (*mol o*, Fig. 6c), and a medium stained inner zone (*mol i*, Fig. 6b). The
stratum granulosum is profusely sprinkled with fairly large black grains (gran,
Fig. 6a, b). The hilus (*CA4*, Fig. 14) is crowded with black mossy fibre boutons
(see, e.g., Haug, 1967). Terminals of mossy fibre collaterals in the subgranular
zone, shown at bottom of Fig. 6a are smaller than in the mossy fibre layer proper.

In the hippocampus, stratum lacunosum moleculare (*lac*, Fig. 14) is on the
whole pale like an adjacent outer zone of the subiculum. In part of CA1 a very
dark wedge extending out from the subiculum is interposed between the major,
pale, part of lacunosum moleculare and the stratum radiatum (asterisk, Fig. 14;
lac, Figs. 5b, c). Stratum radiatum shows medium staining density in CA3 and
in most of CA1 (*rad*, Fig. 5). The mossy fibre layer in CA3 is black (*mf*, Fig. 14)
due to its large, well stained boutons. The pyramidal layer is completely unreac-
tive in CA3 near fascia dentata, but contains fine grains in the rest of CA3 and
especially in CA1. These grains tend to assume an apical position within individual
pyramidal cells (arrows above *pyr*, Fig. 5a). As mentioned above, a pericellular
localization of these granules cannot be excluded.

An outer zone of the molecular layer in the subiculum is pale, as mentioned,
while an inner zone and the cell layers are very dark.

Layer I of the presubiculum (*ps*, Fig. 14) is homogeneously and weakly stained
and is sharply delimited from the subiculum. In area 29e (right arrow, Fig. 14),
the parasubiculum (*pa*, Fig. 14), and the entorhinal area (*em* and *el*, Fig. 14) only
an outer part of layer I is weakly stained. The width of this pale zone is typical
of each area, as is the density of staining in layers II, III, and IV. Layers V and
VI, on the other hand, are more uniformly stained throughout these areas. It is
of interest that particularly intense staining occurs in lamina externa of area 29e
and of 49a (arrows, Fig. 14) and in layer II of area 28 (its lateral part, *el*, Fig. 14).
Special note should also be taken of the sharp delimitation and usually lighter
staining of layer IV in area 28 (its medial part, *em*, Fig. 14). Such sharp interlaminar borders are not found between the deeper layers in any other cortical
area. The border between grey and white matter, however, is more diffuse than
in the neocortex.

The *pyriform cortex* (or primary olfactory cortex, Pigache, 1970), partially
shown in Figs. 19–25, has a pale superficial zone within layer I, continuous with
that in the anterior olfactory nucleus. Details concerning the width and sharpness of definition of this pale zone may provide additional information on the
subdivision of this cortical area, but will not be dealt with in the present text.
The rest of layer I, together with layers II and III, exhibit strong neuropil
staining. The staining of perikarya is variable, usually negligible in layer II (the
dense cell layer), but more pronounced in the deeper layer.

2. Diencephalon[2]

The particulate staining of neuronal somata (p. 18) shows internuclear differences, only some of which will be mentioned in the following account.

As previously explained, glial-like cells with unstained nuclei, small round perikarya and thin, poorly stained processes (2, p. 21) are scattered through most nuclei and fibre tracts but are particularly numerous within the perivascular tangles of stained glial processes (5, p. 23).

The *globus pallidus* (*gp*, Figs. 21–23) and the *entopeduncular nucleus* (*ep*, Fig. 23) are paler than the striatum and strikingly different from the latter with regard to the finer details of staining. They show the characteristic perivascular patches (5, p. 23; Fig. 8a, c) and the occasional staining of fibre bundles (6, p. 23).

The small glial-like cells (2, p. 21) are abundant as is evident from Fig. 8a and c (horizontal arrows). Neuronal somata are stained, although they are not visible in the illustrations.

The *pineal body* (*pi*, Fig. 31) has medium density. In the medial *habenular nucleus* (Fig. 24; *ham*, Fig. 25) the densely packed perikarya show a strong staining which contributes more than that of the neuropil to the total staining. The lateral nucleus (Fig. 24; *hal*, Figs. 1, 25) is on the whole pale. However, a dark patch of perivascular stain borders and infiltrates the fasciculus retroflexus (Figs. 1, 25).

The *dorsal thalamus* (Figs. 1–3, 22–27) is in general weakly stained, but there are differences between areas with only a uniform, fine grain impregnation of the neuropil and other areas with a moderate amount of perivascular staining. Perikarya and capillaries are stained throughout.

Within the *anterior group* (Fig. 23) the anterodorsal (*tad*), and particularly a lateral part of the anteroventral nucleus (*tav*), show moderate intensification of the neuropil staining, while the anteromedial nucleus (*tam*) is pale and diffusely delimited from other medially placed nuclei.

The *lateral nucleus* (*tl*, Figs. 2, 24) shows a marked intensification of the uniform, fine grained staining of the neuropil when compared to the medial and intralaminar nuclei. It was not attempted to determine the posterior extent of this nucleus, nor accordingly, the detailed relation between Timm- and Nissl-architecture at its posterior pole (see Figs. 24–27).

A rounded pale area with slight neuropil stain (Figs. 23–25) corresponds roughly to the *midline and intralaminar* nuclei (Powell and Cowan, 1954a), and the *dorso-medical* nucleus. The distinct posterior border of this area is revealed by sagittal sections (Figs. 1–2) and horizontal sections (Fig. 40a–f). Some midline nuclei show an increased density of the fine grained stain (not visible in the present figures), and within the medial nucleus there regularly occurs an area of perivascular impregnation (*tm*, Figs. 1, 24).

At rostral levels most of the *ventral nucleus* seems to be located within the medial pale area (*tv*, Fig. 23). Further caudally almost the entire ventral nucleus (*tv*, Fig. 25), contains scattered perivascular patches. A similar, weaker stain is

---

2 The following works, in particular, were consulted for the identification of nuclei in the brain stem of the rat: Gurdjian (1927); Crosby *et al.* (1943), particularly Gillilan (1943); Valverde (1962, 1966); Zemann and Innes (1963); König and Klippel (1963); Wünscher *et al.* (1965); Kovac and Denk (1968; mouse brain).

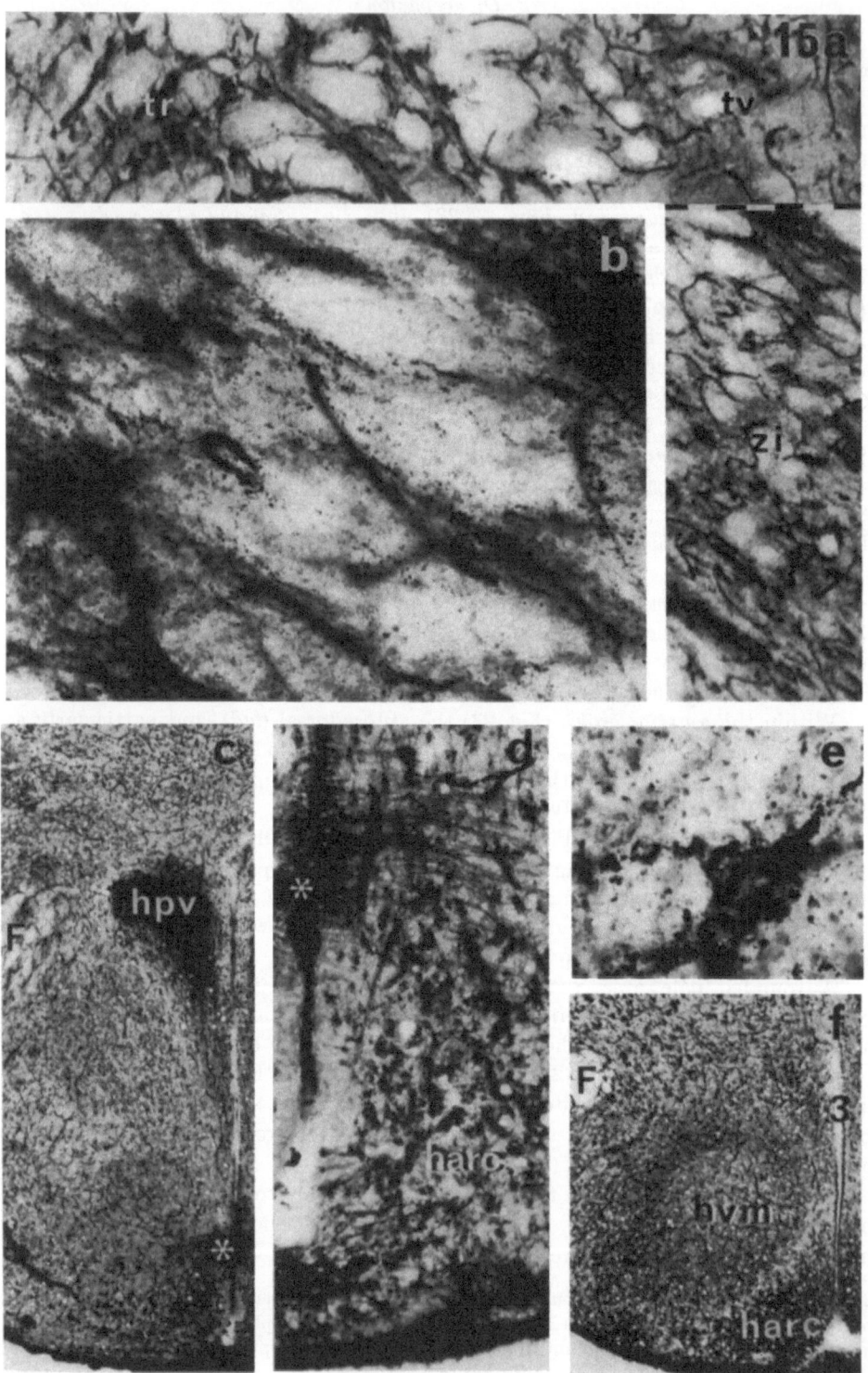

Fig. 15a—f

found within the *geniculate bodies* (*cgld, cglv, cgm*, Figs. 26, 27, and 29). The large perikarya of the *reticular nucleus* stain particularly strongly in contrast to its pale neuropil (*tr*, Figs. 3, 23, 24, 15a).

The *subthalamus* (Figs. 23–25) is delimited from the adjoining nuclei of the dorsal thalamus by virtue of a slightly increased staining of the neuropil. This stain is typically perivascular posteriorly towards the mesencephalic reticular formation (Fig. 15b, *zi*, Figs. 15a, 24, 25), but is more even anteriorly (*zi*, Fig. 23). The *subthalamic nucleus* is distinguished as an area with more numerous and distinctly granulated perikarya (*subt*, Figs. 2, 24).

The *hypothalamus* (Figs. 21–25), blending dorsally with the subthalamic area, has a uniform finely grained stain in the neuropil (Figs. 23, 15c, f), broken only by the largest fibre bundles. Only in the anterior part of the lateral hypothalamic region (*hl*, Fig. 22) does the patchy perivascular stain appear, merging with that of nucleus entopeduncularis, globus pallidus and the lateral preoptic region.

The *medial hypothalamus* displays several internuclear variations in staining of neuropil and particularly of perikarya. Among the most conspicuous features are the very dark *paraventricular* and *supraoptic* nuclei (*hpv, hso*, Figs. 22, 21). Their large perikarya are densely crowded with granules and the neuropil stain is slightly enhanced (*hpv*, Fig. 15c). Profuse granulation of perikarya is also apparent in the *suprachiasmatic* nucleus (*hsc*, Fig. 21). The *arcuate nucleus (harc,* Figs. 23, 15f) is packed with small cells (Fig. 15d) the perikarya of which are filled with particularly large, irregular black particles (not illustrated at higher magnification). The processes of these cells are incompletely stained, which precludes a further comparison with the "spider cells" described by Bleier (1971) as unique for the arcuate nucleus. The *ventromedial nucleus*, on the other hand, is demarcated as an oval area with decreased staining of both perikarya and neuropil, surrounded by a diffuse slightly darker zone (cross, Figs. 22, 23; *hvm*, Fig. 15f). Further internuclear differentiation may be seen in the illustrations.

The anterior hypothalamic and medial preoptic regions (unlabelled, Fig. 21) have a similar density and texture of staining to the greater part of the medial hypothalamus just described. Faint gradients are seen both within these areas and where they blend with the septal area and with a ventral zone of the lateral preoptic region, containing the diagonal band nucleus (see substriatal grey, p. 30).

The *mamillary nuclei* (*m*, Figs. 25, 26) show strongly reacting perikarya, a diffuse neuropil stain, and perivascular patches. Differences in staining could be

Fig. 15a—f. Details from the diencephalon. a) × 112. Nucleus reticularis thalami (*tr*), nucleus ventralis thalami (*tv*) and zona incerta (*zi*). Along the stippled line 4.5 cm of the print was cut out. b) × 450. Zona incerta, anteroposterior level approximately as in Fig. 24. Scattered black particles and small perivascular patches of impregnation. c) × 28. From the hypothalamus. Note uniformity of neuropil stain as compared with patchiness in Fig. 15a and b. d) × 112. Larger magnification of infundibular region with nucleus arcuatus (*harc*) to show its small cells with heavy staining of perikarya and little staining of processes. Note strong impregnation of the smooth basal extensions of ependymal cells in the lateral wall of the third ventricle (at asterisk) and the ventral wall of the infundibulum. e) × 1120. Cell bodies are stained throughout the hypothalamus. The one shown here was selected more or less at random from the medial hypothalamic region, immediately ventral to the fornix in c. f) × 28. Nucleus ventromedialis (*hvm*) surrounded, or encroached upon, by a zone of slightly enhanced neuropil stain

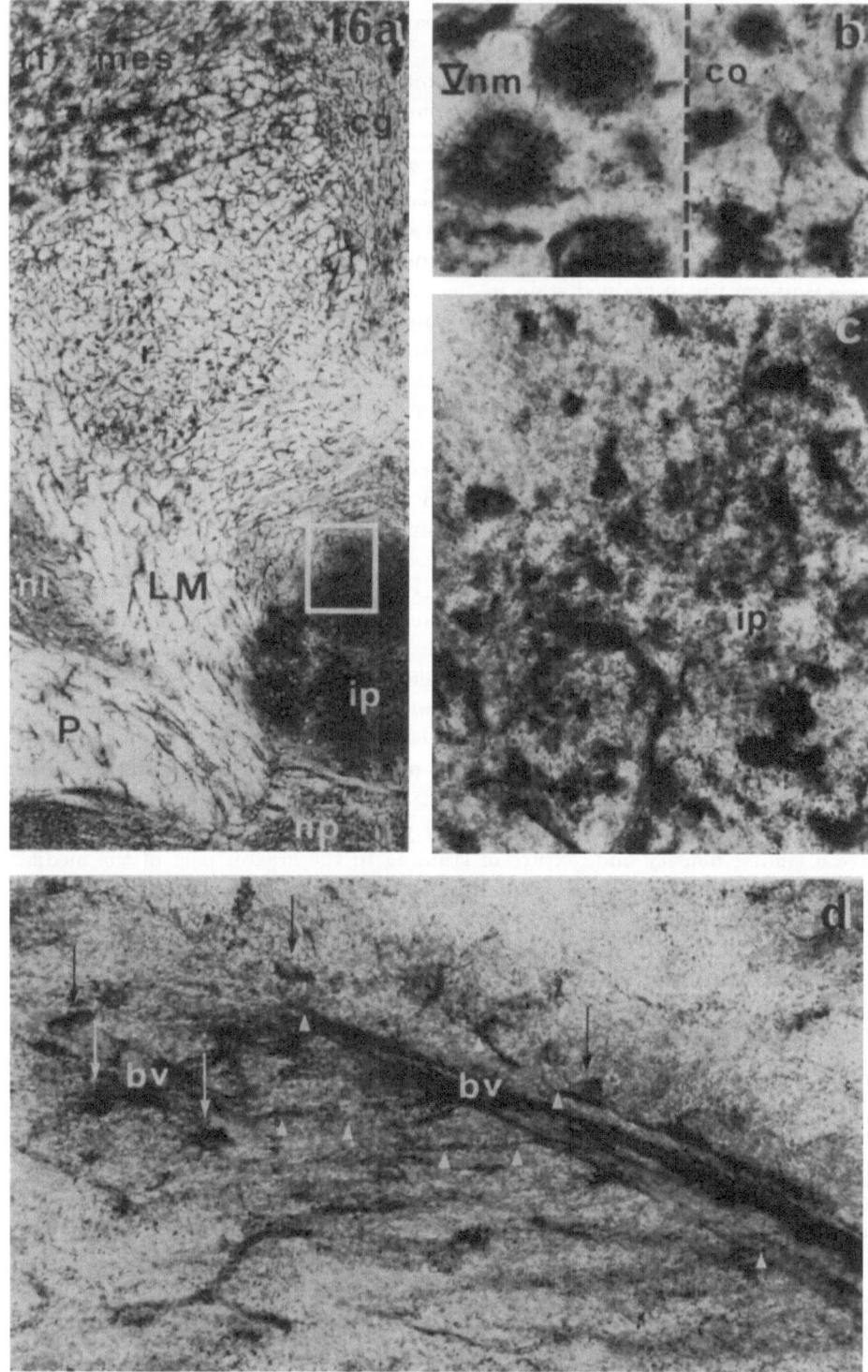

Fig. 16a—d

seen within the mamillary complex but were not further studied since, in the present material, they appeared somewhat variable and did not suggest any immediate correlation with cytoarchitectonics or connections (Powell and Cowan, 1954b; Guillery, 1956, 1957).

3. Mesencephalon

In the *tectum* (Figs. 29–33) perikarya and neuropil are stained, the latter fairly strongly, showing conspicuous perivascular patches (5, p. 23). Lamination in the superior colliculus is faintly revealed due to pale fibre bundles (Fig. 29). The stain in the tectum continues unchanged into lateral *tegmental* areas (*mes*, Figs. 29–30). The border of this large, rather strongly stained, area against the diencephalon is distinct in sagittal (Fig. 1) and horizontal sections (Fig. 40a, c) as already mentioned. In frontal sections a similarly distinct lateral border is seen (Figs. 26–27). This border has not been definitively correlated with cytoarchitectonic features, but probably corresponds to the lateral limit of the *pretectal region* (*pt* in present Figs. 27, 40g)[3].

The *central mesencephalic grey* (*cg*, Figs. 29, 30, and 16a) is usually delimited from the areas just described by a lack of both perivascular staining and coarser fibre bundles. A conspicuous intensification of staining in perikarya and neuropil is displayed by an area of considerable rostrocaudal extent, containing subdivisions (Morest, 1961) of the *dorsal tegmental nucleus* (*dt*, Figs. 1, 31, 32, 40e, f). It shows some internal differentiation which partly reflects cytoarchitectonic features of adjacent Nissl sections. The *laterodorsal* nucleus, including the *locus coeruleus* (Crosby and Woodbourne, 1943), features only slight staining of neuropil and perikarya (*co*, Figs. 31, 32, and 16b). The *ventral tegmental nucleus* (*vt*, Fig. 30) is distinguished by its stained perikarya and so is the *nucleus interstitialis* (Cajal) (*in*, Fig. 27).

Fig. 16a—d. Mesencephalon. a) × 28. The reticular formation at upper left shows perivascular patches of impregnation. One typical patch is shown at higher magnification in d. The central grey matter (*cg*) has a more uniform impregnation. In and around the red nucleus (*r*) there is a virtual absence of neuropil impregnation. Nucleus interpeduncularis (*ip*, window further enlarged in c) has a heavy staining. b) × 450. Large round perikarya of mesencephalic trigeminal nucleus filled with cytoplasmic granules. Some neuronal perikarya in the locus coeruleus are stained, although the staining of somata on the whole is less conspicuous than in many adjacent areas (cp. Fig. 31) (4 cm of the print was cut out along the stippled line.) c) × 450. From area approximately indicated by rectangle in a. The dark impregnation in nucleus interpeduncularis (*ip*, to the right) consists of scattered granules as well as glial cells with the appearance described in text under 2, p. 21. The micrograph does not show the finest visible granules in the neuropil. d) × 450. From the reticular formation. Perivascular patches of impregnation containing small black glial cells (arrows). Note "thread-like" appearance of the other impregnation in these patches (at arrow heads and elsewhere)

---

3 The deeper-lying nucleus, marked with asterisks in Fig. 40c, d (horizontal sections) and Figs. 27, 40 g (frontal sections) is also included in the more strongly stained area medial to the border. It seems to be larger and to extend farther basally than the nucleus pretectalis profundus of Bucher and Nauta (1954) or the nucleus pretectalis anterior of Lund and Webster (1967) and Siminoff et al. (1967), but may fit well with nucleus pretectalis anterior of Scalia (1972). The identification of individual nuclei in the posterior thalamic/pretectal group of cat was discussed recently (Heath and Jones, 1971; Jones and Powell, 1971).

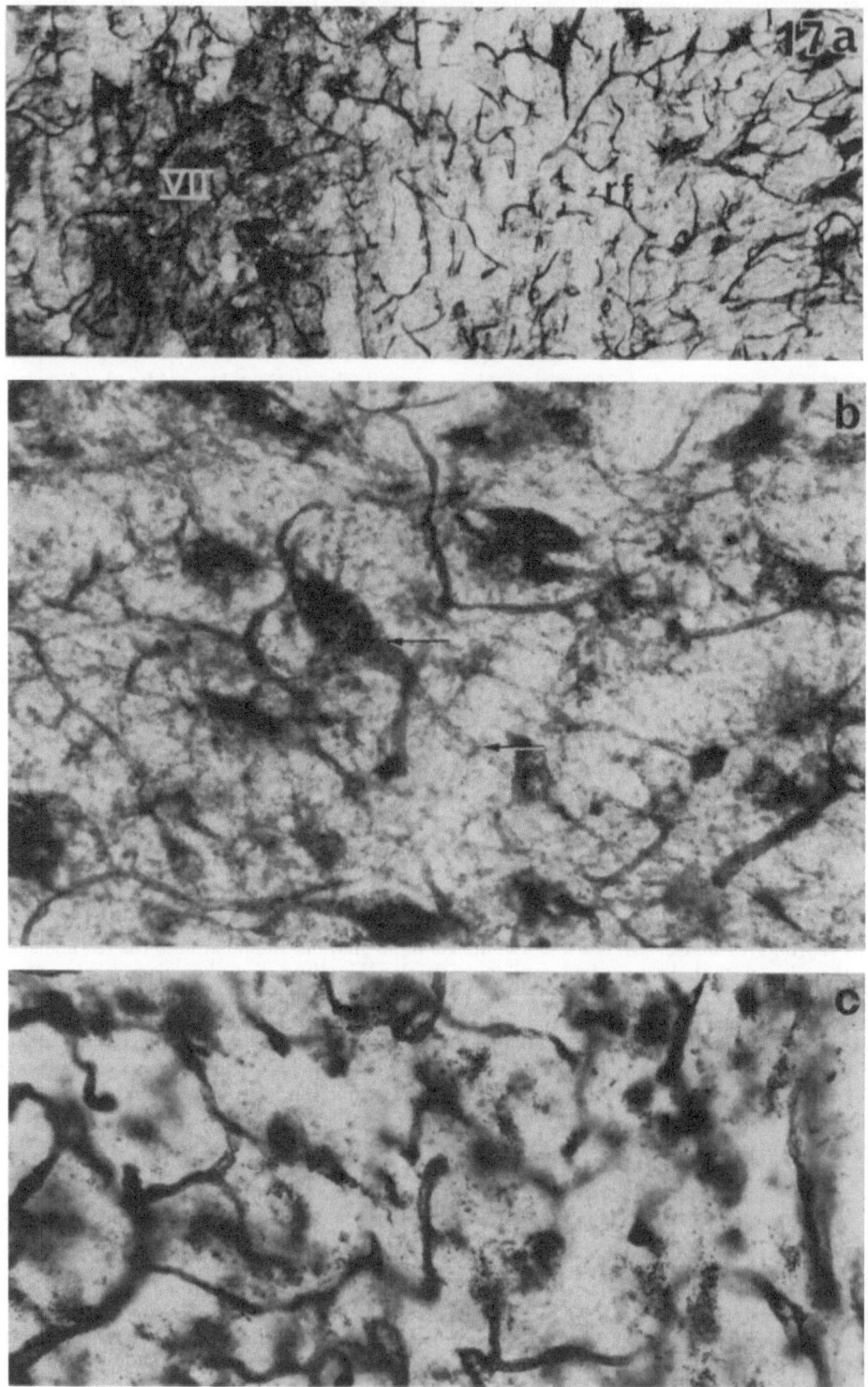

Fig. 17 a—c

The large perikarya of the *mesencephalic nucleus* of the trigeminal nerve (*Vnm*) are crowded with black granules, and thus easily identified even at low magnification (Figs. 16b, 31).

The *red nucleus* is entirely devoid of neuropil stain but its perikarya contain large granules (*r*, Figs. 1, 27, 28, and 16a). In effect, the red nucleus forms the center of a rounded, diffusely delimited area which occupies most of the ventral tegmentum between the medial longitudinal fascicle, the substantia nigra and the interpeduncular nucleus.

At the base of the mesencephalon, extending into the diencephalon, is another somewhat diffuse, pale area (*avt*, Figs. 25, 26). It extends from the interpeduncular and mamillary nuclei medially, in between the medial lemniscus and the substantia nigra laterally. Caudally it is limited by the substantia nigra and the medial lemniscus; rostrally it merges with the lateral hypothalamic region. It will include the *area ventralis tegmenti* of Tsai.

Substantia nigra (*ni*, Figs. 25–27, 16a), pars reticulata, shows a patchy stain of medium density and is somewhat diffusely delimited. Perikarya of the pars compacta are unstained.

The *interpeduncular nucleus* (*ip*, Figs. 27, 16a, c) is darkly stained and—particularly dorsally—sharply delimited. The stain is located in neuronal somata, in small glial-like cells (*2*, p. 21) and in the neuropil. The previously described perivascular staining accounts for at least part of the neuropil stain and further surrounds vessels that leave the dorsal aspect of the nucleus to course through an area including the *nucleus centralis superior* (*cs*, Figs. 1, 28, 29).

4. Pons and Medulla Oblongata

The *reticular formation* is particularly lightly stained as seen at survey magnifications (*rf*, Figs. 30–36). This is due to the presence of numerous unstained fibre bundles and, more significantly, to a lighter staining of the intervening neuropil (Figs. 17a) than found in other locations, e.g., the mesencephalic tectum and dorsolateral tegmentum. The patchy stain surrounding vessels is sparse here (and in the pons and medulla oblongata in general). There may be a slight mediolateral gradient of increasing density of the neuropil stain, but no other gradients reminiscent of differences in connections (Brodal, 1957; Valverde, 1962) nor any borders corresponding to the cytoarchitectonic limits (Meessen and Olszewsky, 1949; Brodal, 1957; Valverde, 1962). Of the three cerebellar projection nuclei,

Fig. 17a—c. From the pons. a) × 112. Staining of perikarya and neuropil in the facial nucleus (*VII*). Neuropil stain somewhat uneven but no prominent perivascular patches are seen. In adjacent medullary reticular formation vessels and neuronal perikarya are stained. b) × 300. Medullary reticular formation. The micrograph does not fully reveal the scattered granules in the neuropil. Stained dendrites, one of which is clearly focussed and indicated by arrows. Capillary stain dominates the picture. Perivascular patches are absent. c) × 450. Nucleus reticularis tegmenti pontis. Virtual absence of neuropil staining in general and of perivascular impregnation of the type shown in a and b. Particulate staining of neurons *reticularis lateralis* shows, at most, a slight intensification of staining, which permits no distinction of limits intra- or internuclearly. The *paramedian reticular nucleus* (Brodal, 1953) cannot be distinguished in Timm sections, but the *reticularis tegmenti pontis*, distinct in Nissl sections, is vaguely discernible on the basis of a virtual lack of staining of the neuropil (*rt*, Fig. 28). Its perikarya are stained, however (dotted cells, Fig. 17c). The raphe nuclei are indistinguishable from their surroundings. The perikarya and proximal dendrites of the giant cells in the medial part of the reticular formation are particularly densely filled with quite large, round, black granules (Fig. 17b).

When compared with the reticular formation, various other nuclei show slight to moderate intensification of the staining of neuropil or perikarya or both. Considering *motor cranial nerve nuclei*, the *dorsal vagal nucleus* (*X*, Fig. 37) and the *hypoglossal nucleus* (*XII*, Figs. 36, 37) are clearly revealed by enhanced staining of the neuropil and a rather fine grained staining of perikarya. The *oculomotor* (*III*, Fig. 29) and *trochlear nuclei* have distinct granulation of perikarya, but otherwise merge with the moderately stained background. The *Edinger-Westphal nucleus* is hardly discernible against the overlying central grey. The neuropil of the *trigeminal motor nucleus* (*V*, Fig. 30) and of the *facial nucleus* (*VII*, Figs. 17a, 30) stains stronger than the adjoining reticular formation. Both nuclei are fairly distinctly delimited from the reticular formation and, but for the existence of intervening fibre bundles, indistinctly delimited from the trigeminal sensory nucleus (*V*, Fig. 30). The stain is localized both to neuropil and perikarya (Fig. 17a). The latter are somewhat more conspicuous in the trigeminal than in the facial nucleus. The perikarya of the *nucleus ambiguus* are more heavily stained than neighbouring cells, but the nucleus is otherwise unremarkable.

The *posterior column nuclei* (*p*, Figs. 37, 38) show an intermediate degree of staining of neuropil and perikarya throughout their extent, including the compact rostroventral cell group of Valverde (1966) (asterisk, Fig. 38) and the external cuneate nucleus.

Among the *sensory cranial nerve nuclei* the spinal (*Vs*) and main (*Vp*) sensory *trigeminal nuclei* are intermediately stained and confluent (Figs. 30, 33–37). In a lateral zone of the spinal nucleus, corresponding to the substantia gelatinosa, the neuropil stain is slightly intensified (Fig. 38).

The *nucleus of the solitary tract* (*sol*, Figs. 36, 37) shows an intermediate staining of perikarya and neuropil comparable to, e.g., the hypoglossal nucleus. It is noteworthy for the distinct delimitation of its neuropil dorsally, medially and ventro-medially, where there is a cell poor border zone (more apparent in adjacent Nissl-sections) that exhibits the medium staining density of the neuropil within the nucleus.

In the *ventral cochlear nucleus* (*cv*, Figs. 30, 31) virtually no staining of the neuropil is found, but there is conspicuous granulation of somata. Conversely the *dorsal* cochlear nucleus (*cd*, Figs. 31–35) has a rather strong patchy staining of the neuropil, and less prominent granulation of many somata. The molecular layer stains weakly and evenly, with medium density, thereby resembling the molecular layers of the cerebellum or the fascia dentata.

The *medial* and *superior vestibular nuclei* merge completely in Timm stained sections (*v*, Figs. 33–35), showing intermediate staining of neuropil and strong granulation of perikarya, while the neuropil between the fibre bundles in the *spinal* nucleus is a little darker (*vs*, Figs. 34 and 35). Granulation of perikarya is less prominent here. The *lateral* vestibular nucleus (Fig. 31; *vl*, Figs. 32, 33), on the other hand, displays very little staining of its rather sparse neuropil, while the giant perikarya abound with black, round and quite large granules and thus resemble the giant cells of the medial reticular formation.

The *inferior olivary* complex (*oi*, Figs. 33, 34, 36) is distinctly delimited due to intermediate staining of perikarya and neuropil. No internal differentiation reflecting the diversity of connections is seen. The *superior olivary* nuclei (*os*, Fig. 29) show a similar staining, while in the medially adjacent *nucleus of the trapezoid body* (*ct*, Fig. 28, 29) stain is restricted predominantly to the perikarya.

Other larger nuclei, or areas, with a similar intermediate staining of neuropil and perikarya are the *nucleus commissuralis* (*comm*, Fig. 38) in the caudal part of the medulla (here the perikarya are rather heavily stained), the *pontine grey* (*np*, Fig. 27), the *parabrachial nuclei* (surrounding *PCS*, Figs. 30, 31), and the *nuclei lemnisci lateralis* (*ll*, Figs. 28, 29). Within the latter nuclei there is a strong staining of the neuropil, divided by large pale fibre bundles.

5. Cerebellum

The cortex (Fig. 18a) appears rather uniform throughout its rostrocaudal and transverse extent (Figs. 31–38). The molecular layer is lightly stained. It has a similar density and appearance as, e.g., the outer third of the molecular layer of the fascia dentata and, at higher magnifications, the stain is partly resolved into discrete particles (*mol*, Fig. 18b) as previously described. A few larger black particles are found, mainly associated with perikarya. The Purkinje cell perikarya show a diffuse yellow staining with superimposed black granules (*pu*, Fig. 18b), while the departing dendrites are indistinguishable from other components of the molecular layer. Immediately above the Purkinje cell layer conspicuous aggregates of large black granules tend to be arranged perpendicular to the cortex (arrows, Fig. 18b). They probably represent Bergmann glia as noted by Timm (1961). Similar but smaller accumulations of granules are found at more superficial levels of the molecular layer.

The granular layer is intermediately stained. At higher magnifications it is profusely dotted (*gr*, Fig. 18b). Finer details will be unmentioned here.

The cerebellar nuclei show intermediate staining of neuropil and perikarya (*cn*, Figs. 18a, 34–37).

6. Spinal Cord

Within grey matter, stain occurs in perikarya and neuropil (Fig. 39). The density of the latter is generally rather low, but increases gradually in the dorsal direction towards a zone of small cells apparently corresponding to Rexed's (1954) laminae I–III in the cat. The staining of perikarya is most easily recognized in cells of intermediate and large size and is seen throughout the grey matter.

White matter stains similarly to that in other regions of the central nervous system.

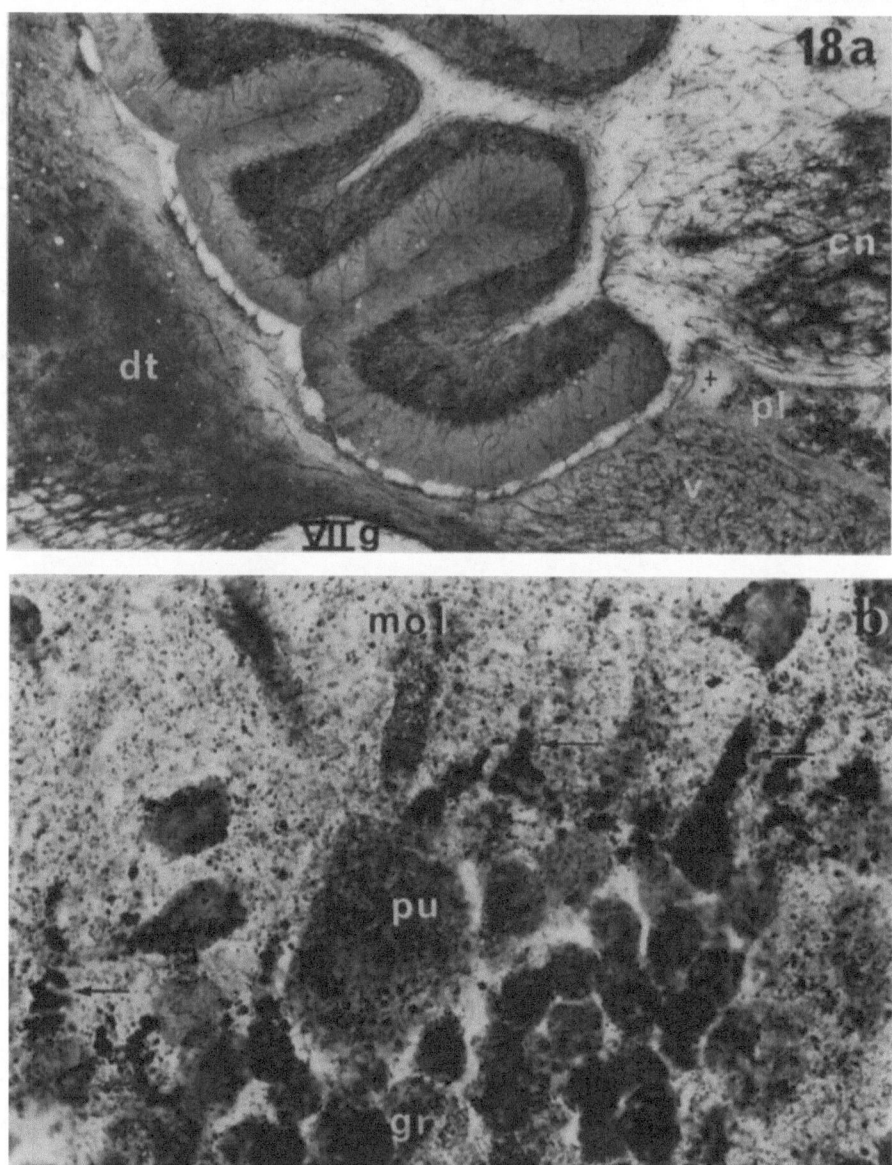

Fig. 18. a) × 35. Cerebellum and adjoining floor of fourth ventricle. From section corresponding closely to Fig. 1. Note diffuse staining within the fourth ventricle (at cross, adjacent
to pale part of the choroid plexus, *pl*). b) × 1120. 10 micron cryostat section counterstained
with thionin. Granules in Purkinje cells (*pu*) represent Timm stain. Note cluster of dark
granules arranged more or less perpendicular to the cortex, possibly representing Bergmann
glia (arrows). Other large particles associated with granule cells. Smaller grains dispersed
in granule cell (*gr*) and molecular (*mol*) layers. Shrinkage artefacts are evident around granule
cells and the Purkinje cell

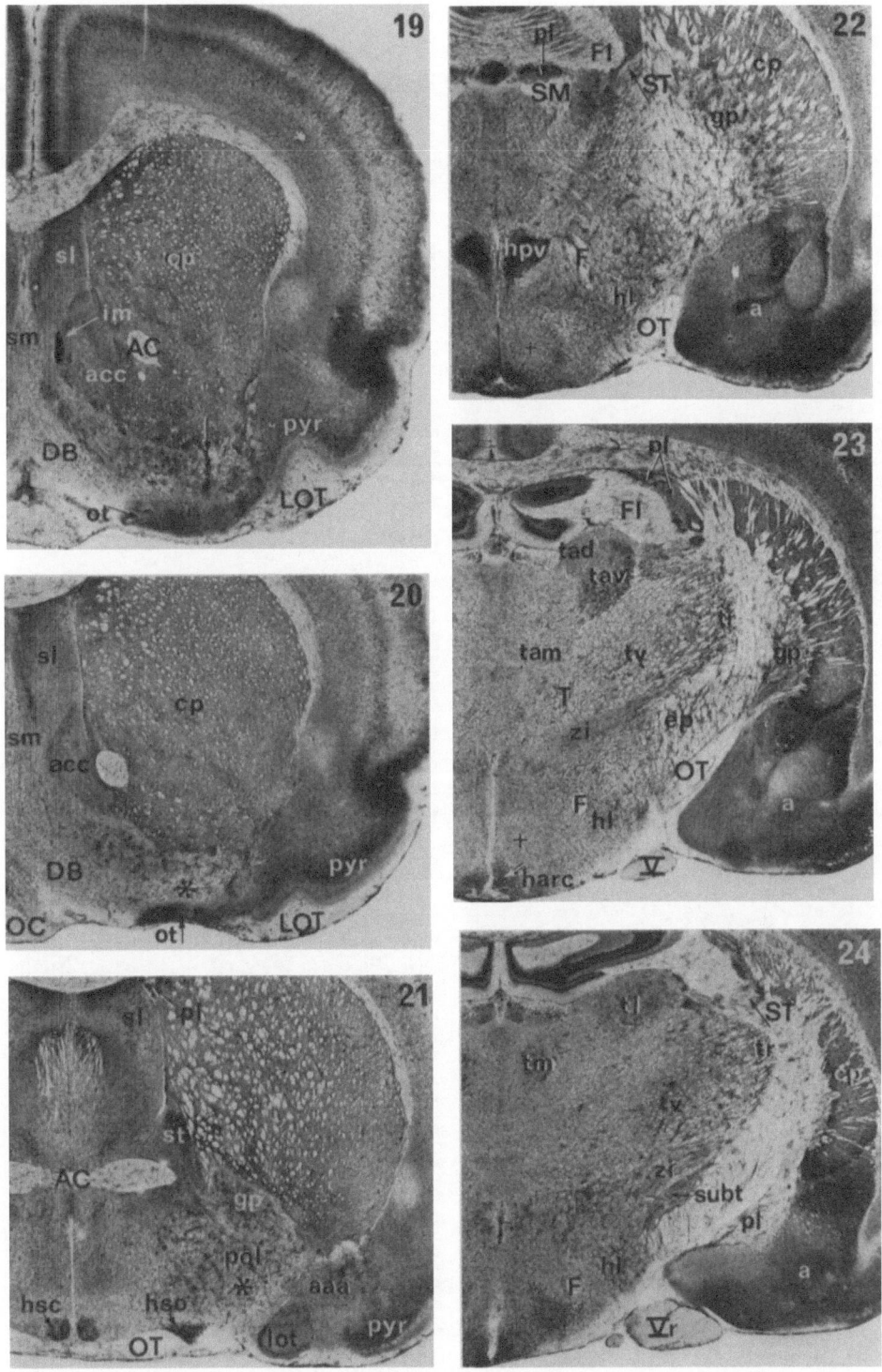

Figs. 19—24. Frontal series × 8.6. 40 micron cryostat sections, stained with Timm's method. For abbreviations, see p. 7. Asterisks in Figs. 20—21, see text p. 30. Cross, Figs. 22—23 in nucleus ventromedialis hypothalami. For further explanation of the figures, see descriptions of individual regions

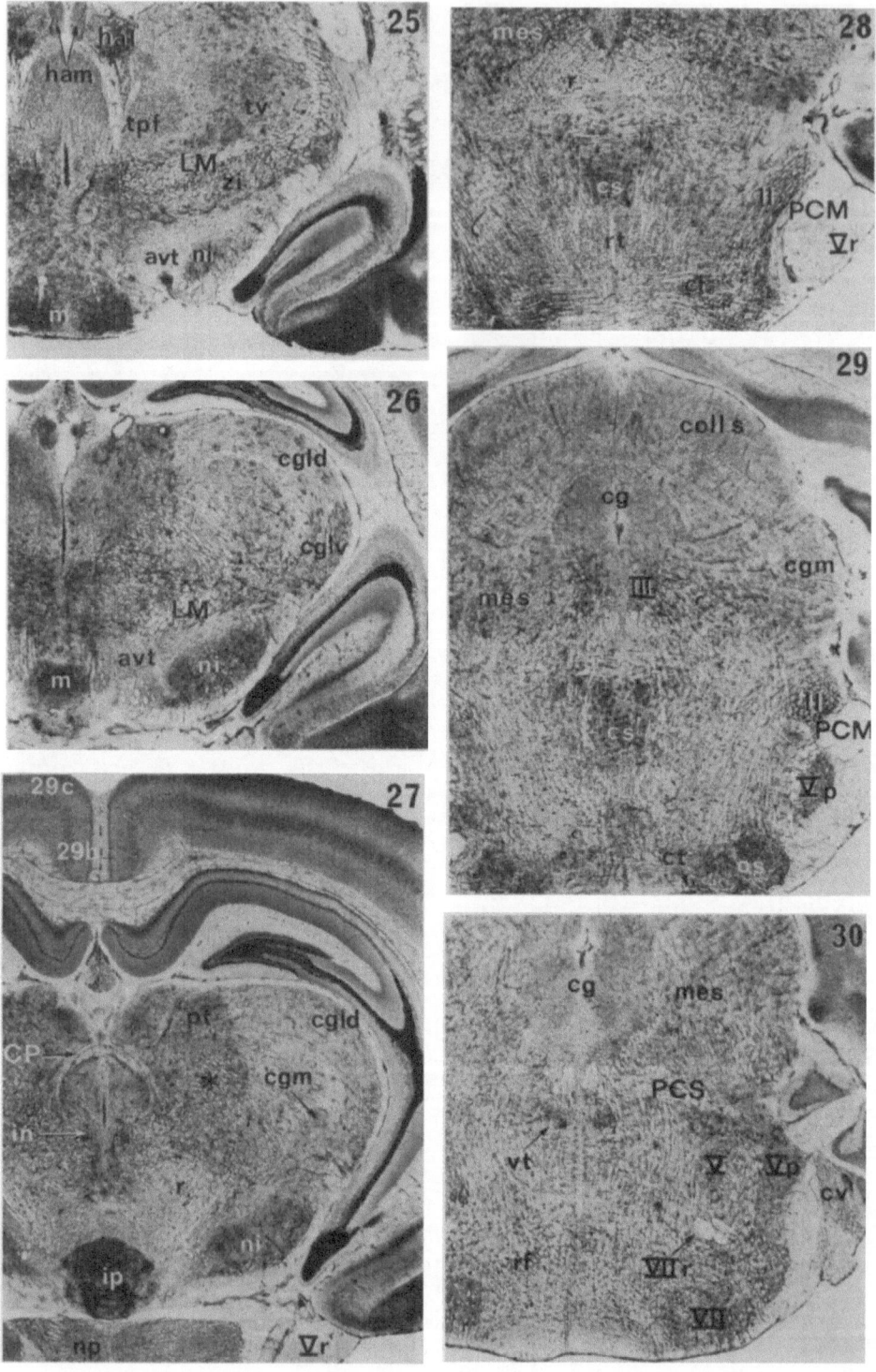

Figs. 25—30. Frontal series × 8.6. 40 micron cryostat sections, stained with Timm's method. For abbreviations, see p. 7. For further explanation of the figures, see descriptions of individual regions

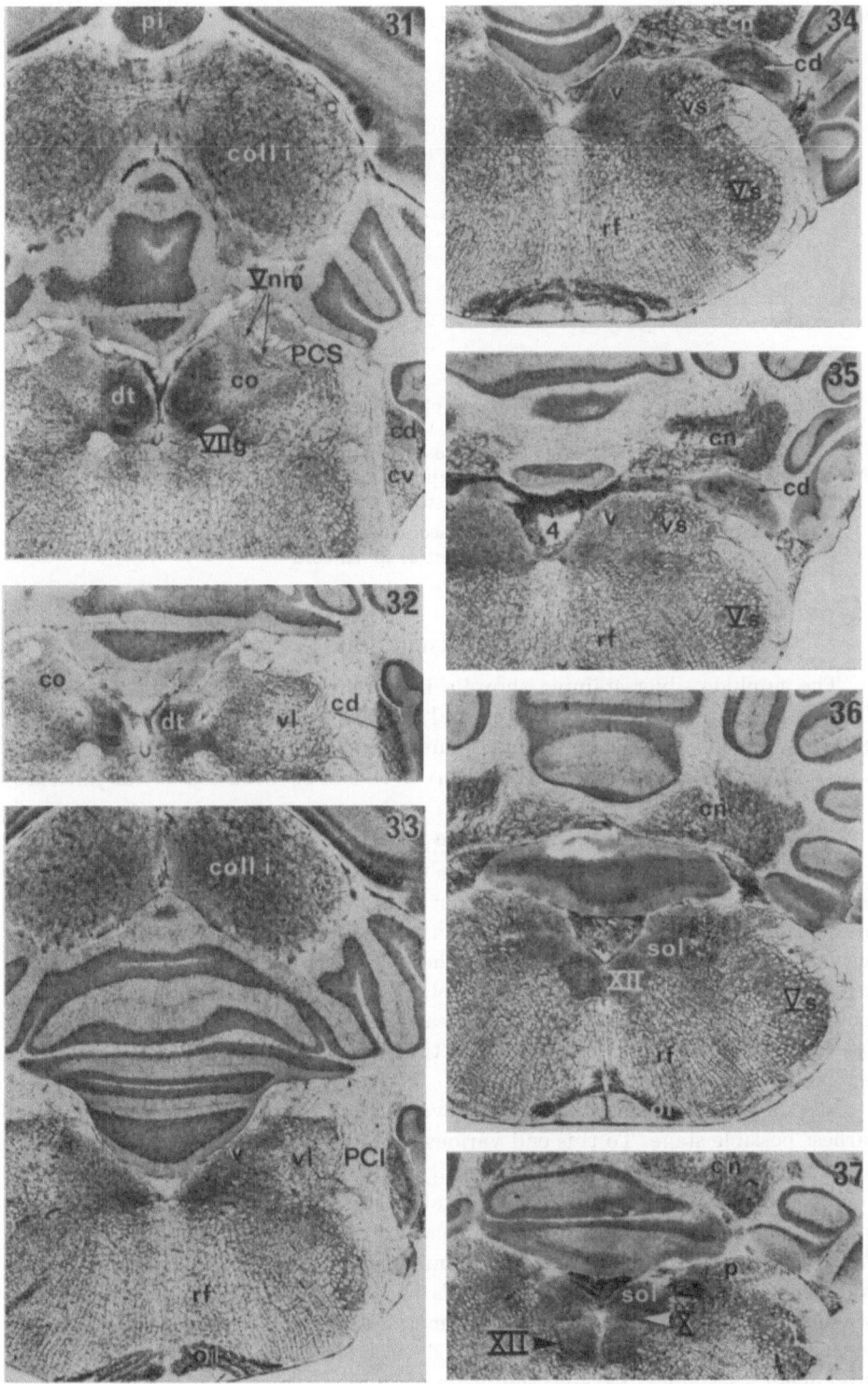

Figs. 31—37. Frontal series × 8.6. 40 micron cryostat sections, stained with Timm's method. For abbreviations, see p. 7. For further explanation of the figures, see descriptions of individual regions

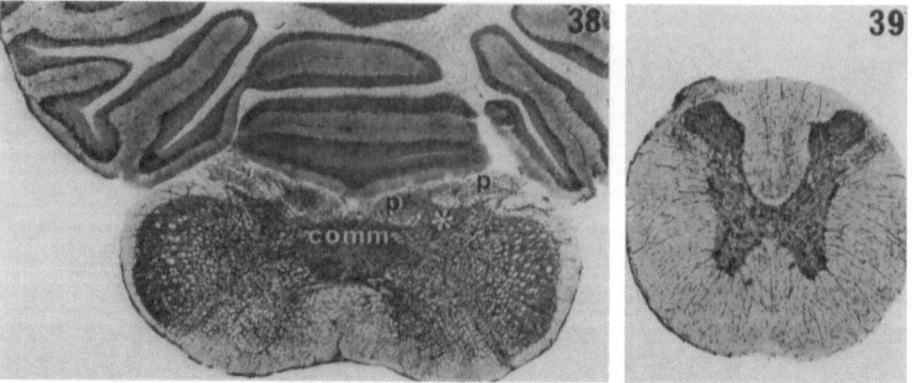

Fig. 38. Frontal series × 8.6. 40 micron cryostat sections, stained with Timm's method.
For abbreviations, see p. 7. For further explanation of the figures, see descriptions of
individual regions. (Asterisk, see text p. 42)

Fig. 39. × 14. 40 micron cryostat section stained with Timm's method,
Thoracic segment of spinal cord

IV. Discussion

The sulphide silver staining shows a high degree of cytological and regional
differentiation throughout the rat central nervous system. The meaning of these
patterns in chemical and functional terms should be analyzed in further experimental work, but some of the problems involved can be discussed at this juncture.

A. The Sulphide Silver Method

This method was introduced by Timm (1958b) and Voigt (1951, 1959) and has
been widely used for the visualization of "heavy metals" in tissue sections. In
principle it involves sulphide precipitation of the metals within the tissue, sectioning, and a subsequent visualization of the metal sulphides by physical development. (In the present context, heavy metals should be taken to mean transition
metals, group IIb metals and other heavy metals. That semimetals, such as
arsene, are also shown with Timm's method was demonstrated by Voigt, 1959
and Voigt and Jonsson, 1961.)

Loss of metals from the tissue is prevented by treating with sulphide at the
earliest possible stage. To this end various procedures have been applied: Simul-
taneous fixation and sulphide treatment in 70% ethanol saturated with H_2S
(Timm, 1958b; Voigt, 1951, 1959); fixation in Carnoy's solution with added
sodium sulphide (Koudousek, 1963); treating native tissue with H_2S gas in a
moist chamber (Timm and Neth, 1959), immersion in ammonium sulphide (Brunk
and Brun, 1972), or perfusion of animals with sodium sulphide as used in the
present investigation. The latter three methods permit cryostat sections to be
prepared, a procedure which has proved superior to paraffin embedding and
subsequent sectioning. Varying the mode of sulphide treatment seemed to effect
minor differences in the relative stainability of neuronal perikarya, glia and neuropil
in general.

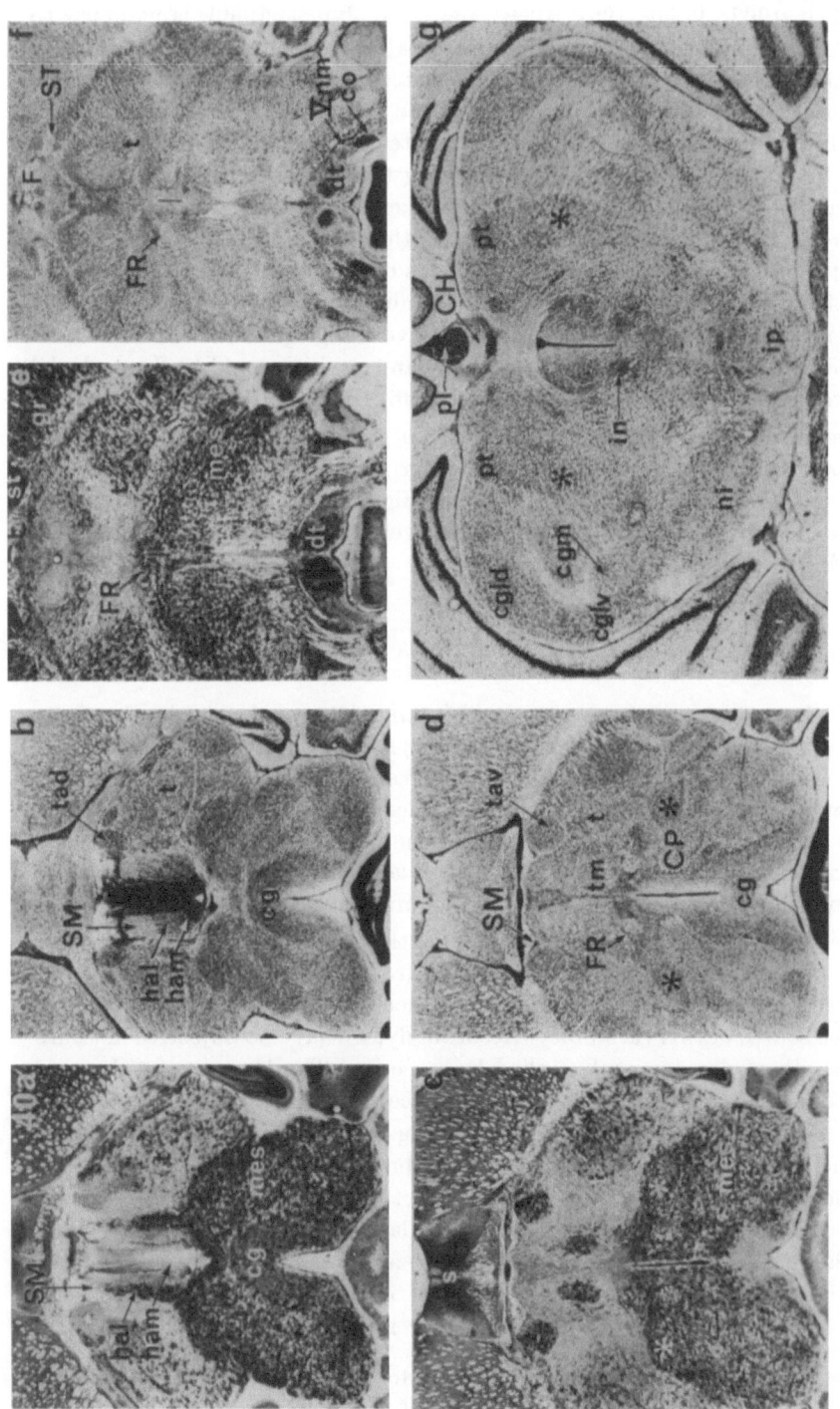

Fig. 40a—g. To show the border between strong Timm staining in the mesencephalon and weaker staining in the diencephalon, and its relation to cytoarchitectonic features. Cell group indicated with asterisk in c, d, g: See text p. 39 (footnote). Other labelling, se list p. 7. a—f) × 5.3. 40 micron horizontal cryostat sections of pairs of adjacent sections (a and b, c and d, e and f) stained with Timm's method and with thionin. g) × 8.6. 40 micron frontal thionine stained cryostat section adjacent to Timm-stained section shown in Fig. 27. Abbreviations, see list p. 7

The staining solution, or physical developer (Liesegang and Rieder, 1921; Timm, 1958b, 1962; Voigt, 1951, 1959; Mees and James, 1966), is assumed to work on the principle that metal sulphides catalyze reduction of silver ions by hydroquinone. Elementary silver is then deposited on the metal sulphides in the tissue. To prevent this reaction from taking place instantaneously throughout the staining solution, gum arabic is added as a "protective colloid". Furthermore pH is lowered by adding an acid or buffer lowering the concentration of negatively charged quinone which is believed to be the active reducing agent[4]. Ambient temperature and lighting are also important for the speed with which the solution decays and the sections stain. The interrelations of these various parameters and their combined effect on the histochemical staining are not known in details. It would seem that a "good" developer should have a high potential for reduction of silver ions but be effectively inhibited in a manner which could be "unlocked" by the metal sulphide precipitates (Querido, 1948).

The present developer was adopted because it gave a stronger and more widespread impregnation of the rat brain than other formulae tried. This is also the impression gathered by comparing the present figures with most of the illustrations given in previous papers on sulphide silver staining of brain tissue (see, however, McLardy, Figs. 7, 8, 1963; 1964).

B. Variations in the Results

The staining pattern in *forebrain neuropil* (and in the molecular layers of the cerebellar cortex and the dorsal cochlear nucleus) is remarkably constant when the present procedures are used. Sometimes, however, there is less than the usual contrast between heavily and lightly stained zones within neuropil of the cerebral cortex due to a diffuse yellow colouration of the normally pale zones (and concurrently of white matter). In the absence of any positive indications to the contrary this should probably be regarded as an unspecific "fog".

As already explained, it is necessary to time the development individually for each batch of slides in order to achieve the desired overall staining intensity. It is most reasonable to assume that the development procedure and not biological factors is the source of this variability. Accordingly, we have no objective measure for the strength of development applied to a section. The best we can do is to regard the over all staining density in the telencephalon as an indication of this parameter. When this is done there seems to be a slight quantitative variation in the stainability of some pale zones in the forebrain such as the outer and inner third of the molecular layer of fascia dentata, the molecular layer of the presubiculum or the outermost part of the molecular layer of other cortical areas. In particular, the outer stained zone in the dentate molecular layer seems to require stronger development to be visualized in some series than in others. (A similar impression is had for the molecular layer of the cerebellar cortex.)

---

4 The "protective" effect of gum arabic seems likely to be attributable to the complexing of silver ions by suitable groups on the polysaccaride or other molecules in this natural product. The high (0.2 M) concentration of citrate could also contribute to the binding of silver ions.

This could mean that the concentration of stainable substances in these zones approaches the limit of detection, giving methodological variations greater importance here than in other regions, or it could reflect biological variation of some kind.

The *neuropil in the brain stem*, particularly the presumed glial processes, also seemed to vary in reactivity from one series to the next.

The staining of *neuronal perikarya in the forebrain* was not consistent, being virtually absent throughout some series and prominent in others that had been developed to about the same degree. *Neuronal perikarya in the brain stem*, on the other hand, seemed to be less variable in this respect, being in general strongly stainable.

With regard to the variable staining of neuronal somata, and of neuroglia, it is pertinent to mention that a decreased staining of these structures can be deliberately induced by using very brief sulphide perfusion (1–2 minutes), by lowering the concentration of sulphide in the perfusate, or by prolonged storage of the cryostat sections in alcohol before they are developed (unpublished observations). Different types of neuronal somata may not be equally susceptible to this influence[5]. The spontaneous variations in staining of perikarya, glia and brain stem neuropil could perhaps in the light of these effects be interpreted as due to insufficient standardization of the sulphide perfusion, but further experiments are needed to evaluate this possibility.

A pertinent question is whether the staining pattern varies in relation to sex or age. The present material was not designed to investigate this systematically, but included adult rats of both sexes weighing from 150 to 300 grammes. The staining of telencephalic neuropil seemed constant but some age-dependant differences within the other components of the total sulphide silver pattern cannot be excluded. In particular the perivascular staining (5, p. 23) often appeared more profuse in younger animals. In this connexion it may be mentioned that immature rat brains show a particularly strong staining of glial cells.

Nutritional or genetic factors may conceivably influence the staining pattern The present procedure is probably sufficiently standardized to allow the detection of any conspicuous differences between experimental groups although it is not suited for exact quantitation as discussed below.

C. Chemical Interpretation of the Staining

Numerous studies show that the sulphide silver method can in fact reveal toxic amounts of metals accumulating in organisms or tissue cultures (Voigt, 1951, 1959; Voigt and Jonsson, 1961; Timm, 1962; Timm *et al.*, 1966a, b; Brunk and Brun, 1972; and others). Similarly, staining is found in cells or tissues where metals are normally present as shown by other histochemical reagents, particularly dithizone, or by chemical analysis.

It should be considered, however,

1. whether other substances than metals may be stained in the present material,

---

5 The solvents involved in paraffin or plastic embedding have a similar effect on the stainability of neuronal somata, neuroglia and vessels to prolonged postfixation of cryostat sections.

2. whether the reaction product reveals the *in vivo* localization of the stainable substance,

3. whether all heavy metals present are revealed,

4. to what extent it is possible to differentiate between various heavy metals, or different metal compounds, and

5. whether a quantitative interpretation of the staining intensities is feasible.

Ad 1. Argyrophilic substances are said to cause precipitation of silver in some tissues without the intervention of sulphide treatment. Such "primary germs" (Voigt, 1951, 1959) may represent metal sulphides formed from exogeneous metals, but may—a priori—also be of non-metallic nature, for instance free sulfhydryl groups (see Brun and Brunk, 1970). This possibility was excluded in the present material by developing sections from brains which had not received any sulphide treatment. Such sections were unstained.

Sulphide treatment might create non-metallic reducing groups in the tissue, e.g. by the breaking of disulphide bonds. But this apparently is not a significant source of artefacts in the central nervous system, since Brun and Brunk (1970) found that the histochemical pattern with a method for sulphydryl groups is unaffected by previous sulphide treatment and bears no resemblance to the present sulphide silver pattern (Brun and Brunk, 1970). It should be noted, however, that because a different sulphide treatment and stronger development was used in the present study than by Brun and Brunk, their observations are not strictly relevant for the present material, especially as regards the neuropil staining.

In the specific instance of the hippocampal mossy fibre boutons, combined evidence from spectrophotometry (Maske, 1955), autoradiography (von Euler, 1962) and atomic absorption spectrophotometry (Hu and Friede, 1968) indicates that the stainable factor is in fact a metal, more specifically zinc. Furthermore, fair correspondence was noted between the sulphide silver pattern and the intravital dithizone stain within the amygdala (Hall *et al.*, 1969). For other central nervous regions experimental evidence on the nature of the argyrophilic germs created by sulphide treatment is sparse, although several transition and group II b metals are known to be present in all parts of the central nervous system (for references see below). It has been found that intravitally administered dithizone (Haug and Danscher, 1971), diethyldithiocarbamate (Danscher *et al.*, 1973) or oxine (Danscher and Fredens, 1972) block the sulphide silver stainability of the mossy fibre areas and practically all other parts of the telencephalic neuropil. Furthermore, perfusion with a dithizone solution before the sulphide will prevent all sulphide silver staining of the rat brain, an effect which is caused by the dithizone itself and not by the buffer in which it is dissolved (unpublished observations). It is recognized that a treatment with chelating agents may not be inert with respect to non-metallic components of the tissue, but these findings are at least well compatible with the assumption that "heavy" metals form the substrate of most or all of the sulphide silver stain described in the present study.

Ad 2. False positive reactions at any given site could be due to the occurrence of metals not present at that site *in vivo*.

Contamination with metals during the preparative procedures probably does not contribute to the characteristic sulphide silver pattern in the brain, since dithizone, when perfused prior to the sulphide, prevents the staining entirely.

Soluble metal complexes might diffuse prior to capture by sulphide, thereafter being revealed in false locations, or metal sulphides might be relocated during the further procedure. Brunk and Sköld (1967) demonstrated shifting of stainability during paraffin embedding and sectioning. For cryostat sections false positive reactions have not been demonstrated (nor excluded). It seems improbable that the elaborate regional differentiation described above arises through relocation of metals during the preparative procedures. However, the apparent staining of "cerebrospinal fluid" perhaps may arise by diffusion of stainable substance from nearby choroid plexus, and the staining occasionally found within cracks in the sections probably reflects diffusion phenomena.

Ad 3. Metals may well be missed with the sulphide silver method, even if they are reactive in inorganic spot tests (Timm, 1962; Brunk *et al.*, 1968).

The sensitivity of the method is one potentially limiting factor. Concerning this, Feigl (1958) states the lowest concentration of silver detectable in his spot test to be $1:10000000$ ($= 0.1$ µg pr. ml), and the smallest amount detectable at this concentration, $0.005\,\gamma$ ($1\,\gamma = 1$ µg). Similar data were not given for other metals. The recommended procedure was to place a drop of the silver solution on a filter paper, which is then exposed to sulphide and stained by physical development. The sample volume corresponding to the above amount and concentration would be 50 µl, producing a large spot on the filter paper. In the histochemical procedure the limits of detectability must be strongly influenced by factors such as size and distribution of organelles, section thickness, and the resolution of the microscope procedure used. Obviously, the degree of development is particularly important. Realistic model experiments permitting the evaluation of such factors have not been reported, so Feigl's figures should be used with caution. For comparison, nonetheless, recent investigations on the metal content of central nervous regions indicate that the concentration of manganese, copper, zinc and iron ranges from 0.2 to more than 50 µg/g wet weight, depending on the region and the type of metal (Thompson, 1961; Cumings, 1961; Courville *et al.*, 1963; Schmidt and Manhart, 1968; Hu and Friede, 1968; Wong and Fritze, 1969; Harrison *et al.*, 1968; O'Neal *et al.*, 1970; Crawford and Connor, 1972). Similar values were found by Matsuba and Takahashi (1970) for subcellular fractions of brain tissue. A priori, the concentration of a given metal may well be a total of values for different substances binding it, some of which could be below the limit of detectability of the sulphide silver method or not stained for other reasons.

Another way that metals may be missed is by conversion (oxydation) of the sulphide, which will abolish the argyrophilia and increase the solubility of the metal (Brunk and Sköld, 1967). This may be the reason for the gradual decline and eventually complete loss of stainability in neuronal perikarya, glia, choroid plexus, and vessels, which occurs when the sections are stored in alcohol or water, prior to development (p. 51). It is remarkable that the pattern of reactivity within the telencephalic neuropil is not changed by such treatment.

It has also been suggested that easily diffusible metal complexes could escape the sulphide fixation (Timm, 1962; Pihl and Falkmer, 1967).

Finally it is most important that many metal complexes in the tissues are probably not available to the sulphide under the conditions used. Examples of this may be found in the heme bound iron of erythrocytes and mitochondria, since the sulphide silver staining of these structures is negligible. The differentiated regional staining pattern, including virtually unstained neuropil, conforms with the idea that only a few metalloenzymes (Vallee and Wacker, 1970) or other biological metal complexes (Johnson and Seven, 1961) contribute significantly to the staining pattern. Chemical analyses of macro- and microsamples are needed to elucidate these problems. In addition, model experiments may give useful indications of the sensitivity of the sulphide silver method towards specific biologically important metal complexes.

Ad 4. To differentiate between various heavy metals and metal complexes the following experimental approaches may be taken:

Timm and Neth (1959), Timm (1961, 1962) and others, recommend stepwise dissolution of metal sulphides based on differential solubility in acid, metal-complexing or oxidizing solutions. In none of these reports were procedures and results specified in full practical detail. Bog and Stegner (1954), Voigt (1959), Kaltenbach and Eger (1966) and Brunk *et al.* (1968) reported equivocal results of such tests. These findings as well as rather obvious theoretical considerations imply that solubility tests for metal sulphides may only be relied upon after their significance has been defined with independant methods for the biological system under consideration—as stated clearly by Bog and Stegner (1954). Stegner and Fischer (1957) suggested, as an alternative to the dissolution of metal sulphides, that pH and other conditions during the initial stage of sulphide treatment be adjusted to achieve selective precipitation of groups of metals. Independant validation of these procedures also appear necessary. Therefore, similar experiments were not included in the present study. However, as mentioned above, neuronal somata, neuroglia and vessels (but not telencephalic neuropil) lose stainability when sulphide treated material is stored in ethanol or physiological saline and this is probably due to solubilization of metal sulphides. Furthermore, preliminary investigations have confirmed that acids remove most of the argyrophilic germs created by the sulphide treatment, those in neuropil included. These phenomena may now be investigated in detail using as a base the standardized procedures and "normal" staining pattern described in the present report.

It may, in addition, be worthwhile to try to chelate metals selectively with various agents administered by intravital injections or by perfusion *prior to* the sulphide treatment (since a chelating agent may act quite differently within living, dead and sulphide treated tissue). It was mentioned above that preperfusion with dithizone removes all sulphide silver stainability from the brain, whereas intravital injections of dithizone (Haug and Danscher, 1971) or diethyldithiocarbamate (Danscher *et al.*, 1973) affects telencephalic neuropil more strongly than somata, neuroglia or vessels. In preliminary experiments intravitally injected 2-2'-dipyridyl prevented much of the staining in somata and neuropil while leaving the hippocampal mossy fibre system apparently untouched. Thiosemicarbazide (100–200 mg pr. kg, intravitally) had no effect on the subsequent sulphide silver staining. Such experiments, carried out systematically, may aid in classifying different components of the staining pattern.

It must be remembered that besides the stability constants of metal complexes measured *in vitro*, several factors may confer selectivity on interactions between exogeneous ligands and tissue-bound metals (Albert, 1961; Eichhorn, 1961; Malmström, 1961; Vallee and Wacker, 1970). Accordingly, direct chemical analyses appear indispensable for determining the nature of the Timm stainable metal[6]. It may be helpful to carry out parallel analyses of "normal" and experimentally altered material, however, including experiments of the type just indicated.

As has already been indicated, probably only a fraction of the metal compounds are revealed with the present method. This should simplify the interpretation of the staining. High spatial resolution of the methods that are combined (electron microscopy, subcellular fractionation, regional dissection of stained and unstained layers) will also facilitate the task of equating different components of the sulphide silver stainable substance with individual metals and well defined metal compounds.

Ad 5. Obviously, a quantitative interpretation of the relative staining densities is not yet feasible. We may, nonetheless, assume that a difference in darkness between individual stained granules of similar size reflects a difference in their concentration of stainable substances. A difference in the time needed to reach identical densities would similarly reflect concentration differences. A pertinent example is provided by the particles, within neuronal perikarya and glial cells, which are about 1 micron in size and yet stain completely black within 20 to 30 minutes; compared to the much larger hippocampal mossy fibre boutons which become faintly visible at 20 minutes and turn black only at 50 to 60 minutes. It is reasonable to conclude that the concentration of stainable metals is considerably higher within the granules of neuronal and glial perikarya than in the hippocampal mossy fibre boutons.

A comparison of individual stained elements in the telencephalic neuropil with the large mossy fibre boutons reveals no such convincing differences in time taken to reach comparable densities. The mossy fibre boutons appear darker, but that may be an effect of their larger size.

The density of a given region obviously depends on the fraction of tissue volume occupied by stained particles and the staining intensity of the particles.

D. The Cellular Localization of the Stain

On the basis of the present light microscope data the stained structures were arbitrarily grouped as neuronal somata, neuroglia and neuropil in general. For a definitive determination of the fine structural localization of the stain, electron microscopy and subcellular fractionation are required. Some comments on these questions should, however, be made.

In general the present elaborate, regional staining pattern implies selective staining of cellular and subcellular structures as well. It is also noteworthy that electron microscopy of various non-nervous cells and organs in sulphide silver material has indicated an association with membrane bound organelles in many cases (Müller and Geyer, 1965, 1970; Okamoto and Kawanishi, 1966; Phil, 1967;

---

6 The possibility that other histochemical methods for heavy metals, already existing (see e.g. Pearse, 1972 for a survey) or yet to be developed, may provide supplementary information cannot of course be disregarded.

Phil and Falkmer, 1967; Scheuer et al., 1967): The electron dense precipitate in these studies consisted of discrete granules scattered within or along the surface of the stained organelles and cells (see also p. 58).

1. Neuronal Perikarya

Brun and Brunk (1970), using the light microscope, reported a good correlation between the distribution of sulphide silver stained granules and lysosomes in the neocortex and hippocampus. The variation in staining between somata of different types and in different regions invites further studies along this line. It should be emphasized that the present cryostat material—even including the 2–3 micron sections—does not show whether all sulphide silver stained granules associated with perikarya are intracellular. Thus, the stained dots within the dentate granule cell layer and particularly those in the apical part of the hippocampal pyramids cannot be definitively classified in this respect.

2. Neuroglia

The classification of neuroglia, based on light microscopy, is still controversial as is evident from recent reviews by Polak (1965) and Cammermeyer (1966).

Most recent electron microscope studies support the classical distinction of three major morphological types of glia (Blinzinger and Hager, 1964; Mugnaini et al., 1967; Holländer et al., 1969; Stensaas and Stensaas, 1968a, b; Vaughn and Peters, 1968; Torvik and Skjørten, 1971), although a few have failed to reveal clear evidence for microglia (Maxwell and Kruger, 1966; Kruger and Maxwell, 1966; Caley and Maxwell, 1968). In any event, the histogenetic derivation and developmental potentialities of microglia are still under discussion (Vaughn and Peters, 1968). The list of sulphide silver stained glial patterns given above (section III-B-3) is meant to be purely descriptive and provisional. It cannot be used for a definitive classification into major types and subtypes of glia, but may be valuable by indicating a chemical heterogeneity of glial cells, which could be further investigated using other methods.

The cells, indicated in paragraph 1 (section III-B-3), with the round or fusiform perikarya and well impregnated, irregular, processes, have the appearance of microglia; although some of them have rather large perikarya and long processes.

The cells tentatively grouped as a separate category under 2 might be either microglia, for some reason less heavily stained, or incompletely impregnated oligoglia. The latter interpretation fits their round form, sparse cytoplasm and apparently thin processes (compare e.g., Stensaas and Stensaas, 1968a, b), but would imply that only a fraction of the oligoglial cells in the central nervous system are stained. Both alternatives raise the question why sulphide silver stained cells of this appearance are especially abundant in restricted areas of the brain stem.

The cells grouped under 3 by virtue of their weak stainability and usually smooth processes, present the typical picture of astroglia; although some weakly stained cells did show more irregular processes.

The cells listed under *4* (characterized by only a few strongly reactive particles in their perikarya and proximal processes) are probably, in part, weakly stained versions of the cell types already discussed. In this connexion it is relevant that Bergmann glia in the cerebellum and astroglial-like cells in many fibre tracts indeed show this kind of staining and that some nuclei within the oligoglial rows in white matter are also surrounded by similar particles. In the latter instance, the fact that there are far more oligoglia than aggregates of Timm positive granules in these rows implies that either these Timm-stained particles do not lie in oligoglia or, again, that cells in the oligoglia group differ in reactivity.

Processes of cells in the three first groups described here, were seen to connect with the walls of vessels, as has been observed for all major types of glia (Cammermeyer, 1966). Cells appearing to lie directly on the vessel walls, singly or in rows, might be termed pericytelike pending electron microscopic studies; or it could be suggested that they are oligoglia. Cammermeyer (1960) showed small round perivascular (oligoglial) perikarya often tightly apposed to the vessel and forming long rows. The small, round, Timm-stained perikarya seen in the present material (*2*, p. 21) look quite similar.

The patches described under *5* constitute a major part of the staining in many diencephalic regions. Their content of faint strands or threads radiating from the central vessels suggests that glial processes rather than axons, boutons or dendrites are stained. Investigations with other methods are needed to substantiate this.

The regional variation in staining of the ependyma and the choroid plexus was not systematically studied, and no explanation of the variation can be given. In general, it could be due to a partial loss of stainable substance by diffusion (p. 53). Regional differences, however, have also been found in the ependyma and choroid plexus with other methods, including enzyme histochemistry (discussion by Bleier, 1971), rendering true differences in metal content an additional and plausible alternative.

All the questions discussed above concerning the chemical significance of the sulphide silver stain apply to the staining of glial cells. Two further points may be raised here.

First, it could perhaps be discussed whether the homogeneous black staining of glial cells represents a "dark cell" artefact (see Cammermeyer, 1962) due to handling of the sulphide-treated but unfixed tissue prior to freezing. However, the regular occurrence of many characteristic cells in specific locations militates against this suggestion. It is more probable that the intense staining of these cells in fact reflects a particularly high concentration of stainable substances, and that glial cells differ from each other and from neurons with respect to their content of Timm stainable metals.

Second, it is reasonable to ask whether the patches that in some regions surround vessels and individual glial cells are artefactual. The vessel walls in these regions might be so constituted that the perfused sulphide acts particularly strongly in their neighbourhood. This possibility is excluded by the presence of exactly the same staining pattern in unperfused brains which have instead been immersed in sulphide buffer, ammonium sulphide solution or physiological saline saturated with H_2S-gas, or which were treated with H_2S-gas directly (unpublished observations).

It cannot be excluded, however, that perivascular glial perikarya, or their processes, or both, contain a particularly diffusible Timm positive substance which contributes some diffuse stainability to their surroundings.

Concluding, the marked regional differences and distinct borders with respect to sulphide silver stainability of glia, and the apparent differences within morphologically defined types of glial cells, invite further study.

3. Neuropil

a) Telencephalon

The staining of the hippocampal mossy fibre layer, which was the point of departure for the present investigation, proved to be confined to the boutons of the layer, as mentioned in the introduction. It consisted of discrete grains, some 500 Å in diameter, spread diffusely throughout the substance of the boutons while lacking in mitochondria (Haug, 1967; Ibata and Otsuka, 1969). The number of grains in any single thin section of a bouton was surprisingly low in view of the homogeneous, dark appearance of the boutons seen in the light microscope[7].

Electron microscope investigations in progress show that the precipitate in other parts of the hippocampus consists of similar grains which tend to aggregate within membrane bound profiles. Structural damage from the physical developer has so far prevented a complete identification of the stained profiles, however.

The present light microscope findings show that axons or myelin contain at most a minor fraction of the Timm-stainable substance, since white matter and recognizable fibre bundles are pale and the picture in general is entirely different from what is seen with reduced silver methods for axons, or with myelin stains. Similarly, the stain cannot be diffusely distributed within or on the surface of dendrites. Boutons, dendritic spines, glial cell processes and particular organelles within one or more of these structures, or within dendrites, are the remaining possible loci of staining. Individual stained elements frequently resemble boutons in form and size. They are often found to be absent from at least the central part of dendrites. In these instances boutons or spines become the elements most likely to contain the stain.

Additional clues may be found in some details of the laminar pattern in certain cortical areas. Thus, the outer part of layer I in most regions is pale although it contains numerous dendrites ascending from deeper layers. At the subiculohippocampal transition a narrow, heavily stained, zone is interposed between the paler stratum radiatum and the nearly unstained major part of stratum lacunosum-moleculare. The dendrites traversing this well-stained zone inhabit also the neighbouring paler strata. Similarly, in the dark layer II of area 28 L or of the presubiculum no dendritic plexus confined to this layer has been described so far. Finally, the illuminating situation in the fascia dentata should be emphasized. Granule cell dendrites in large numbers intermingled with a few

---

7 Although these grains were about the size of synaptic vesicles, their relation to the latter was not investigated. Nor is there any other evidence on whether the stainable substance is located within, upon or between the synaptic vesicles. It may be significant but hardly conclusive that there were far less grains of precipitate than synaptic vesicles within the mossy fibre boutons.

dendrites of other types traverse the trilaminar molecular layer. No local dendritic plexuses exist that could correspond to the outer and inner darker parts of the layers but still the middle part of the layer is unstained.

According to our present knowledge, these examples of lamination along the course of a dendritic tree are most easily explained by assuming a presynaptic localization of the stain, analogous to the proven example in the case of the hippocampal mossy fibre boutons. It is true that differential histochemical reactivity in different parts of cerebellar dendrites and axons has been shown by Hajós et al. (1969) with a histochemical method for succinic dehydrogenase, but only a gradual decrease of staining intensity in a peripheral direction was seen. The present findings would, if a dendritic localization were accepted, rather imply specific chemical functions within sharply defined segments of the dendritic tree or its spines, possibly localized to the postsynaptic membrane. Analogous conjectures might be made for glial cell processes. Both alternatives appear at present less proable than a localization in boutons. It should again be emphasized that within most individual stained brain fields or single layers probably only a minority of the structures (boutons, spines, synapses) are Timm-positive, as suggested by the variegated regional pattern which comprises several nonreactive or weakly stained synaptic fields.

Concluding, it is evident that the sulphide silver pattern in the neuropil of the hippocampal region correlates extremely well with the pattern of synaptic fields revealed by reduced silver methods (Blackstad, 1956; Hjorth Simonsen, 1971, 1972, 1973; Hjorth Simonsen and Jeune, 1972; Zimmer, 1971). Therefore, whatever the identity and exact localization of the sulphide silver stained substances, they will in this part of the brain obviously prove to have a close functional and structural association with synapses of specific fibre systems. It is reasonable to suspect a similar association within other parts of the forebrain where the stain has the same general appearance.

b) Brain Stem, Cerebellum and Spinal Cord

As previously discussed, a great deal of the staining density in these locations, in particular the patchy perivascular staining, is probably due to impregnation of glial processes. A minor fraction is located within the dendrites of certain neurons, farther out from the somata than is seen in the telencephalon.

With regard to the nature of the stained particles that are distributed evenly throughout parts of the thalamus, large portions of the hypothalamus, the periaqueductal grey, the cerebellar cortex, and elsewhere, no definite suggestions can be made. Nor do the observations favour any special interpretation of the enhanced neuropil stain within the interpeduncular nucleus, the dorsal tegmental nucleus and several cranial nerve nuclei.

E. Timm Staining of Paraffin Sections

Paraffin embedded material has been used in the present study to demonstrate absence of staining within large cortical dendrites. Better preservation of morphological detail was obtained in this way at the expense of a higher risk of dissolving or destroying argyrophilic germs.

The following observations suggest that no significant loss of stainable substance occurred from large dendrites in the paraffin sections as compared to the cryostat sections:

1. Storage (postfixation) of *cryostat sections* in ethanol for several days prior to development does not affect the characteristic neuropil pattern within the telencephalon, suggesting that the stainable substance concerned should resist the solvents involved in paraffin embedding as well.

2. The regional staining pattern of telencephalic neuropil in the paraffin sections resembles that of cryostat sections.

3. In so far as the finer distribution of the neuropil stain in the telencephalon may be observed in cryostat sections it corresponds to that seen in paraffin material: The granular appearance of the stain is very similar, and unstained stripes may be faintly discerned in several cortical regions.

F. Concluding Remarks

1. The Morphological Significance of the Regional Staining Patterns

Any staining which can reveal distinct borders and subareas within the brain is of interest in neurobiological studies, even if its functional significance is at present completely unknown. Adequate delimitation and subdivision of areas are the primary requisite for studies of fine structure, fibre connections, embryonic development, and comparative anatomy, as well as for physiological and chemical studies. The sulphide silver stain deserves general application for its ability to give valuable clues to the definition and subdivision of areas, while demonstrating sharp borders as well as gradual transitions between areae or laminae. Within parts of the mammalian telencephalon useful delimitations have already been obtained, e.g., the septum, olfactory tubercle and substriatal grey, pyriform cortex, amygdala, cingulate cortex and hippocampal region. The staining pattern in the hippocampal region of the rat is presently under detailed study (Haug, 1973). It is likely that comparative studies with Timm's method even in submammalians will prove fruitful.

It is obvious that an understanding of the ultrastructural, chemical and physiological significance of the staining will enhance the value of such morphological analyses.

2. Possible Functional Implications of the Staining

It is too early to make specific suggestions concerning the chemical and functional roles of the stainable substances, but some general considerations may be of interest. Metalloenzymes and other metalloproteins, which are being demonstrated in increasing number (Vallee and Wacker, 1970; Mildvan, 1970), could account for some of the stainability. Therefore it is natural to ask whether any information may be gained from a comparison with other histochemical patterns. Known zinc enzymes for which histochemical methods exist include alkaline phosphatase and carbonic anhydrase. They have not been mapped in detail, but available data do not suggest a significant correspondance with the Timm pattern. Several dehydrogenases are known or suspected to contain zinc, but the Timm pattern, e.g., in the hippocampal region, is not explainable on the basis of published maps of dehydrogenase activity (Mellgren and Blackstad, 1967). Nor does any convincing correspondance emerge from a comparison with the histochemical distribution of other enzymes—irespective of metal content.

It should be emphasized that interaction *in vitro* between trace metals and many biological molecules other than proteins are known (see Johnson and Seven, (1961). However, information concerning the mode of binding and the functions of heavy metals *in vivo* is sparse outside the field of metalloproteins or metal porhyrins.

Considering the staining in *neuronal somata, neuroglia* and *brain stem neuropil* as a whole, a heterogeneous group of subcellular elements is probably involved. If so, the stainable substances in question may have varied functions, perhaps of a general metabolic nature. As mentioned, Brun and Brunk (1970) suggest that lysosomes are the particles stained within neuronal somata. A similar particulate staining is also found in many other cell types throughout the body (Timm, 1958 b, 1962; Timm and Schulz, 1966 b; Voigt, 1951, 1959; Kaltenbach and Eger, 1966; Müller and Geyer, 1965; Brun and Brunk, 1970, and others).

If the staining throughout *telencephalic neuropil* is shown to be in fact associated with specific synapses and located presynaptically—as in the hippocampal mossy fibre system—it will be tempting to suggest that the stainable metals share a common type of function within these synapses, or even that we are dealing with one and the same substance.

In considering whether the stainable metals in the mossy fibre system and other synaptic fields could have, in a sense, more specific "synaptic" functions, the following data and experimental approaches may be noted:

Heavy metals influence various membrane functions (Bowler and Duncan, 1970), and Del Castillo *et al.* (1971) found that heavy metals influence the electrochemical functions of motor endplates on microelectrophoretic application. It has further been suggested that some trace metals, including calcium, magnesium, iron, copper and zinc, could form complexes with neurotransmitters in synaptic vesicles (Colburn and Maas, 1965; Pletscher *et al.*, 1970; Rajan *et al.*, 1971) and influence membrane transport of transmitters and inorganic ions (Maas and Colburn, 1965). Catecholamines were the transmitters considered in these reports and catecholamine terminals distribute according to a different pattern from that of the sulphide silver stainable metals throughout most forebrain areas (see Fuxe, 1965; Fuxe *et al.*, 1968; Blackstad *et al.*, 1967). However, metals might interact with other transmitters in a similar manner.

The rapid bleaching of hippocampal mossy fibre boutons (within 10 to 20 hours) during anterograde axon degeneration (Haug *et al.*, 1971) could be taken to suggest a normally rapid turnover of the metal in these boutons, not inconsistent with the participation in synaptic transmission.

As mentioned, von Euler (1962) showed electrophysiologically that sulphide treatment abolished the transmission in the mossy fibre synapses, presumably by binding the Timm stainable metal. Similar experiments with other ligands are tempting. Fleischhauer and Ohnesorge (1958) showed that intravitally administered dithizone has massive behavioural effects in experimental animals while leaving simpler reflexes intact. Their experiments, although based on crude evaluation, suggested an interference with higher nervous functions due to the binding of metals. As mentioned, the sulphide silver staining throughout the forebrain neuropil is blocked immediately by the dithizone injections (Haug and Danscher, 1971), and diethyldithiocarbamate has a similar effect (Danscher *et al.*, 1973).

Chelating a metal in a particular site by exogeneous ligands perhaps does not always interfere with its normal functions. Thus, diethyldithiocarbamate binds to the copper in uricase but is replaced competitively by substrate and does not inhibit the enzyme (Mahler *et al.*, 1955; and others, cited after Westerfeld, 1961). Furthermore, chelating agents may have effects not related to metal binding or may bind metals not demonstrable with Timm's method. Both are the case with diethyldithiocarbamate which is a sulphydryl reagent and binds the copper in dopamine-β-hydroxylase (probably unstainable with Timm's method), thereby inhibiting noradrenaline synthesis. Nevertheless, is seems possible that binding the Timm stainable substances within forebrain synapses produces a rapid, reversible, behavioural effect as discussed by Danscher *et al* (1973).

It should be worthwhile to screen other chelating agents for effects on the Timm pattern; in particular substances with recognized neuropharmacological activity. Numerous drugs form metal complexes *in vitro*, but little is known concerning the importance of such mechanisms for their actions *in vivo* (Chenoweth, 1956, 1961; Weinberg, 1957; Foye, 1961). Interaction of different drugs with the sulphide silver stainable metals may serve to elucidate the normal functions of these metals and could eventually become of pharmacological interest as well.

The conclusion to be drawn at this juncture is that ultrastructural and direct chemical investigations on the nature of the Timm stainable substances are indispensable for further research on their functions. It is hoped that the present observations may guide the sampling and facilitate the interpretations in such studies.

V. Summary and Conclusions

Timm's sulphide silver method is generally regarded as a sensitive histochemical method for transition metals, group IIb metals, and heavy metals. It has been used frequently both for investigating the localization of metals normally present in various tissues and, in animal experiments, for tracing the distribution of metals administered in toxic amounts. In the present paper detailed practical procedures are described which ensure a reproducible, strong, sulphide silver staining in the central nervous system of the rat. The regional and detailed distribution of the stain is described and problems related to its histochemical interpretation surveyed.

White matter is lightly stainable, some of the stain clearly being located in glial perikarya and processes, and the rest more diffusely distributed. Various fibre tracts differ moderately from each other in reactivity.

Various types of stained glial cells are described. There are clear regional differences in the staining of glia. It is concluded that the present method reveals chemical differences within the major morphological types of glial cells. The ependyma and choroid plexus are stained, as are capillaries and vessels of slightly larger calibre.

Neuronal somata show characteristic reactivities ranging from none to strong with the staining usually confined to granules. Some somata have an additional diffuse background stain.

Within the neuropil sharp borders as well as diffuse gradients between nuclei, areae and laminae exist as further described in the text. Most of the stain is again confined to granules, whose size range varies regionally.

In the telencephalon the staining of neuropil is generally much stronger than elsewhere, and the granules are evenly distributed within a given layer or field. In the cerebral cortex and the amygdala the granules appear to be excluded from dendritic shafts. Occasionally they invest dendritic shafts, suggesting a localization to boutons or spines.

In parts of the diencephalon, including the pallidum, and in the mesencephalon, there are diffuse perivascular patches, containing numerous stained glial perikarya as well as grains and fine strands which may represent glial processes. Other lower centres show a uniform, weak stain in the neuropil.

In the Discussion, sources of artefacts and possible chemical interpretations are dealt with. A major part of the stain is probably due to transition metals, but only some of the transition metal compounds in the tissue are likely to be stained. The exact subcellular location and functional significance of the stain must await further studies. Nonetheless, within telencephalic neuropil the regional distribution suggests that the stainable substances are associated with specific synapses, perhaps being confined to boutons, as is known to be true in the layer of hippocampal mossy fibres. The chemistry of the Timm stainable substances, when determined, must be expected to characterize these fibre systems or synapses *vis-a-vis* others that are unstained.

The purely morphological applications of the sulphide silver method is emphasized. It is a highly valuable supplement to conventional methods for delimiting and subdividing cortical and subcortical grey matter, and may provide a useful way of marking specific fibre systems.

Acknowledgements. This study was carried out in the Institute of Anatomy, University of Oslo, during the last 6 years; and in the Institute of Anatomy, University of Aarhus, during several temporary engagements since 1970. It was supported in part by U.S.P.H.S. Grant NS 07998, which is hereby gratefully acknowledged.

I wish to express my sincere gratitude to professor T. W. Blackstad, head of the Institute of Anatomy B, Aarhus University, for enthusiastic support and thorough criticism of the manuscript.

I am also greatly indebted to professor F. Walberg, head of the Institute of Anatomy, University of Oslo, who has created excellent working facilities, including necessary new equipment and technical assistance.

Professor A. Torvik, Ullevål Hospital, Department of Pathology, kindly commented upon parts of the manuscript, especially the sections on glia.

The expert aid of several technical coworkers of both institutes was indispensable to the completion of the present study. Turid Lindstad prepared the cryostat sections finally used for illustrating the present paper. The final photographic prints were made by Einar Risnes, Berit Branil and Albert Meier, and were mounted and labelled by Nanty Stang Lund. Wenche Sandberg rendered bibliographical assistance. Ingeborg Fridstrøm, Solveig Rasmussen, and Lene Knudsen were mainly responsible for the typing. I am very grateful to them all.

References

Albert, A.: Design of chelating agents for selected biological activity. In: Biological aspects of metal binding (L. A. Johnson, M. J. Seven, eds.). Fed. Proc., Suppl. 10, 137–147 (1961).

Blackstad, T. W.: Commissural connections of the hippocampal region in the rat, with special reference to their mode of termination. J. comp. Neurol. 105, 417–538 (1956).

Blackstad, T. W., Brink, K., Hem, J., Jeune, B.: Distribution of hippocampal mossy fibers in the rat. An experimental study with silver impregnation methods. J. comp. Neurol. 138, 433–450 (1970).

Blackstad, T. W., Fuxe, K., Hökfeldt, T.: Noradrenaline nerve terminals in the hippocampal region of the rat and the guinea pig. Z. Zellforsch. 78, 463–473 (1967).

Bleier, R.: The relations of ependyma to neurons and capillaries in the hypothalamus: A Golgi-Cox study. J. comp. Neurol. 142, 439–464 (1971).

Blinzinger, K., Hager, H.: Elektronenmikroskopische Untersuchungen zur Feinstruktur ruhender und progressiver Mikrogliazellen im ZNS des Goldhamsters. In: Topics in basic neurology (W. Bargmann and J. P. Schadé, eds.). Progress in brain research, vol. 6, p. 99–111. Amsterdam: Elsevier 1964.

Bog, R., Stegner, H.-E.: Versuche mit der physikalischen Entwicklung am tierischen Darm. Acta histochem. (Jena) 1, 29–41 (1954).

Bowler, K., Duncan, C. J.: The effects of copper on membrane systems. Biochim. biophys. Acta (Amst.) 196, 116–119 (1970).

Brodal, A.: The amygdaloid nucleus in the rat. J. comp. Neurol. 87, 1–16 (1947).

Brodal, A.: Reticulo-cerebellar connections in the cat. An experimental study. J. comp. Neurol. 98, 113–154 (1953).

Brodal, A.: The reticular formation of the brain stem. Anatomical aspects and functional correlations. The Henderson Trust Lectures, No XVIII. Edinburgh: Oliver and Boyd 1957.

Brun, A., Brunk, U.: Histochemical indications for lysosomal localization of heavy metals in normal rat brain and liver. J. Histochem. Cytochem. 18, 820–827 (1970).

Brunk, U., Brun, A.: Histochemical evidence for lysosomal uptake of lead in tissue cultured fibroblasts. Histochemie 29, 140–146 (1972).

Brunk, U., Brun, A., Sköld, G.: Histochemical demonstration of heavy metals with the sulfide-silver method. A methodological study. Acta histochem. (Jena) 31, 345–357 (1968).

Brunk, U., Sköld, G.: The oxidation problem in the sulfide-silver method for histochemical demonstration of metals. Acta histochem. (Jena) 27, 199–206 (1967).

Bucher, V. M., Nauta, W. H. J.: A note on the pretectal cell groups in the rat's brain. J. comp. Neurol. 100, 287–296 (1954).

Cajal, S.: Histologie du système nerveux de l'homme et des vértebrés. T. II. Paris: A. Maloine 1911; reprinted Madrid: Instituto Cajal 1955.

Caley, D. W., Maxwell, D. S.: An electron microscopic study of the neuroglia during post-natal development of the rat cerebrum. J. comp. Neurol. 133, 45–70 (1968).

Cammermeyer, J.: Reappraisal of the perivascular distribution of oligodendrocytes. Amer. J. Anat. 106, 197–231 (1960).

Cammermeyer, J.: An evaluation of the significance of the "dark neuron". Ergebn. Anat. Entwickl.-Gesch. 36, 1–61 (1962).

Cammermeyer, J.: Morphological distinctions between oligodendrocytes and microglia cells in the rabbit cerebral cortex. Amer. J. Anat. 118, 227–248 (1966).

Chenoweth, M. B.: Chelation as a mechanism of pharmacological action. Pharmacol. Rev. 8, 57–87 (1956).

Chenoweth, M. B.: Known and suspected role of metal coordination in drug action. In: Biological aspects of metal binding (L. A. Johnson and M. J. Seven, eds.). Fed. Proc., Suppl. 10, 125–129 (1961).

Colburn, R. W., Maas, J. W.: Adenosinetriphosphate—metal—norepinephrine ternary complexes and catecholamine binding. Nature (Lond.) 208, 37–41 (1965).

Courville, C. B., Nussbaum, R. E., Butt, E. M.: Changes in trace metals in brain in Hunting-ton's chorea. Arch. Neurol. (Chic.) 8, 481–489 (1963).

Crawford, J. L., Connor, J. D.: Zinc in maturing rat brain: Hippocampal concentration and localization. J. Neurochem. 19, 1451–1459 (1972).

Crosby, E. C., Woodbourne, R. T.: Discussion of the literature. In: Huber, G. C. Crosby, E. C., Woodbourne, R. T., Gillilan, L. A., Brown, J. O., Tamthar, B.: The mammalian midbrain and isthmus regions. Part I. The nuclear pattern. J. comp. Neurol. 78, 129–534 (1943).

Cumings, J. N.: The chemical pathology of copper. In: Chemical pathology of the nervous system (J. Folch-Pi, ed.). Proc. Third Internat. Neurochem. Symposium, Strasbourg 1958, p. 126–139. Oxford: Pergamon Press 1961.

Danscher, G., Fredens, K.: The effect of oxine and alloxan on the sulfide silver stainability of the rat brain. Histochemie 30, 307–314 (1972).

Danscher, G., Haug, F.-M. Š., Fredens, K.: Effect of diethyldithiocarbamate (DEDTC) on sulphide silver stained boutons. Reversible blocking of Timm's sulphide silver stain for "heavy metals" in DEDTC treated rats (light microscopy). Exp. Brain Res. 16, 521–532 (1973).

Del Castillo, J., Escobar, J., Gijón, E.: Effects of the electrophoretic application of sulfhydryl reagents to the end-plate receptors. Int. J. Neurosci. 1, 199–209 (1971).

Domesick, V. B.: Projections from the cingulate cortex in the rat. Brain Res. 12, 296–320 (1969).

Eichhorn, G. L.: Metal chelate compounds in biological systems. In: Biological aspects of metal binding (L. A. Johnson, M. J. Seven, eds.). Fed. Proc., Suppl. 10, 40–51 (1961).

Euler, C. von: On the significance of the high zinc content in the hippocampal formation. In: Physiologie de l'hippocampe (P. Passouant, ed.), p. 135–145. Paris: Editions du Centre National de la Recherche Scientifique 1962.

Feigl, F.: Spot tests in inorganic analysis, p. 61–62. Translated by R. E. Oesper. 5th Engl. ed. Amsterdam-London-New York-Princeton: Elsevier 1958.

Fleischhauer, K., Horstmann, E.: Intravitale Dithizonfärbung homologer Felder der Ammonsformation von Säugern. Z. Zellforsch. 46, 598–609 (1957).

Fleischhauer, K., Ohnesorge, F. K.: Zur Pharmakologie des Dithizon. Naunyn-Schmiedebergs Arch. exp. Path. Pharmak. 235, 63–77 (1958).

Foye, W. O.: Role of metal-binding in the biological activities of drugs. J. pharm. Sci. 50, 93–108 (1961).

Fuxe, K.: Evidence for the existence of monoamine neurons in the central nervous system. IV. Distribution of monoamine nerve terminals in the central nervous system. Acta physiol. scand. 64, Suppl. 247, 37–85 (1965).

Fuxe, K., Hamberger, B., Hökfeldt, T.: Distribution of noradrenaline terminals in cortical areas of the rat. Brain Res. 8, 125–131 (1968).

Gillilan, L. A.: The nuclear pattern of the non-tectal portions of the midbrain and isthmus in rodents. J. comp. Neurol. 78, 213–251 (1943).

Guillery, R. W.: Degeneration in the post-commissural fornix and the mamillary peduncle of the rat. J. Anat. (Lond.) 90, 350–371 (1956).

Guillery, R. W.: Degeneration in the hypothalamic connexions of the albino rat. J. Anat. (Lond.) 91, 91–115 (1957).

Gurdjian, E. S.: The diencephalon of the albino rat. Studies on the brain of the rat, No 2. J. comp. Neurol. 43, 1–114 (1927).

Hajós, F., Kerpel-Fronius, S.: Electron histochemical observation of succinic dehydrogenase activity in various parts of neurons. Exp. Brain Res. 8, 66–78 (1969).

Hall, E., Haug, F.-M. Š., Ursin, H.: Dithizone and sulphide silver staining of the amygdala in the cat. Z. Zellforsch. 102, 40–48 (1969).

Harrison, W. W., Netsky, M. G., Brown, M. D.: Trace elements in human brain: Copper, zinc, iron and magnesium. Clin. chim. Acta 21, 55–60 (1968).

Haug, F.-M. S.: Electron microscopical localization of the zinc in hippocampal mossy fibre synapses by a modified sulfide silver procedure. Histochemie 8, 355–368 (1967).

Haug, F.-M. S.: Light microscopical mapping of the hippocampal region of the rat with Timm's sulphide silver method for heavy metals. (In preparation 1973).

Haug, F.-M. S.: Blackstad, T. W., Simonsen, A. H., Zimmer, J.: Timm's sulphide silver reaction for zinc during experimental anterograde degeneration of hippocampal mossy fibres. J. comp. Neurol. 142, 23–32 (1971).

Haug, F.-M. S.: Danscher, G.: Effect of intravital dithizone treatment on the Timm sulfide silver pattern of rat brain. Histochemie 27, 290–299 (1971).

Heath, C. J., Jones, E. G.: An experimental study of ascending connections from the posterior group of thalamic nuclei in the cat. J. comp. Neurol. 141, 397–426 (1971).

Hjorth-Simonsen, A.: Fink-Heimer silver impregnation of degenerating axons and terminals in mounted cryostat sections of fresh and fixed brains. Stain Technol. 45, 199–204 (1970).

Hjorth-Simonsen, A.: Hippocampal efferents to the ipsilateral entorhinal area: An experimental study in the rat. J. comp. Neurol. 142, 417–438 (1971).

Hjorth-Simonsen, A.: Projection of the lateral part of the entorhinal area to the hippocampus and fascia dentata. J. comp. Neurol. 146, 219–232 (1972).

Hjorth-Simonsen, A.: Some intrinsic connections of the hippocampus in the rat: an experimental analysis. J. comp. Neurol. 147, 145–162 (1973).

Hjorth-Simonsen, A., Jeune, B.: Origin and termination of the hippocampal perforant path in the rat studied by silver impregnation. J. comp. Neurol. 144, 215–232 (1972).

Holländer, H., Brodal, P., Walberg, F.: Electronmicroscopic observations on the structure of the pontine nuclei and the mode of termination of the corticopontine fibres. An experimental study in the cat. Exp. Brain Res. 7, 95–110 (1969).

Horstmann, E.: Die Faserglia des Selachiergehirns. Z. Zellforsch. 39, 588–617 (1954).

Hu, K. H., Friede, R. L.: Topographic determination of zinc in human brain by atomic absorption spectrophotometry. J. Neurochem. 15, 667–685 (1968).

Ibata, Y., Otsuka, N.: Electron microscopic demonstration of zinc in the hippocampal formation using Timm's sulfide-silver technique. J. Histochem. Cytochem. 17, 171–175 (1969).

Johnson, L. A., Seven, M. J. (eds.): Biological aspects of metal binding. Fed. Proc., Suppl. 10 (1961).

Jones, E. G., Powell, T. P. S.: An analysis of the posterior group of thalamic nuclei on the basis of its afferent connections. J. comp. Neurol. 143, 185–216 (1971).

Kaltenbach, T., Eger, W.: Beiträge zum histochemischen Nachweis von Eisen, Kupfer und Zink in der menschlichen Leber unter besonderer Berücksichtigung des Silber-Sulfid-Verfahrens nach Timm. Acta histochem. (Jena) 25, 329–354 (1966).

Koudousek, R.: Carnoy-Natriumsulfidgemisch als Fixierungs-Mittel bei der Sulfid-Silbermethode nach Timm. Acta histochem. (Jena) 15, 386–388 (1963).

Kovac, W., Denk, H.: Der Hirnstamm der Maus. Topographie, Cytoarchitektonik und Cytologie. 150 pp. Wien-New York: Springer 1968.

Krieg, W. J. S.: Connections of the cerebral cortex. I. The albino rat. A. Topography of the cortical areas. J. comp. Neurol. 84, 221–275 (1946).

Kruger, L., Maxwell, D. S.: Electron microscopy of oligodendrocytes in normal rat cerebrum. Amer. J. Anat. 118, 411–436 (1966).

König, J. F. R., Klippel, R. A.: The rat brain. A stereotaxic atlas of the forebrain and lower parts of the brain stem. Baltimore: Williams and Wilkins 1963.

Leonhardt, H.: Über Ependymale Tanycyten des III. Ventrikels beim Kaninchen in Elektronenmikroskopischer Betrachtung. Z. Zellforsch. 74, 1–11 (1966).

Liesegang, R. E., Rieder, W.: Versuche mit einer „Keimmethode" zum Nachweis von Silber in Gewebsschnitten. Z. wiss. Mikr. 38, 334–338 (1921).

Lohman, A. H. M.: The anterior olfactory lobe of the guinea pig. Acta anat. (Basel) 53, Suppl. 49, 1–109 (1963).

Lorente de Nó, R.: Studies on the structure of the cerebral cortex. I. The area entorhinalis. J. Psychol. Neurol. (Lpz.) 45, 381–438 (1933).

Lorente de Nó, R.: Studies on the structure of the cerebral cortex. II. Continuation of the study of the ammonic system. J. Psychol. Neurol. (Lpz.) 46, 113–177 (1934).

Lund, R. D., Webster, K. E.: Thalamic afferents from the spinal cord and trigeminal nuclei. J. comp. Neurol. 130, 313–328 (1967).

Maas, J. W., Colburn, R. W.: Co-ordination chemistry and membrane function with particular reference to the synapse and catecholamine transport. Nature (Lond.) 208, 41–46 (1965).

Mahler, H. R., Hübscher, G., Baum, H.: Studies on uricase. I. Preparation, purification and properties of a cuproprotein. J. biol. Chem. 216, 625–641 (1955).

Malmström, B. G.: Role of metal binding in enzymic reactions. In: Biological aspects of metal binding (L. A. Johnson and M. J. Seven, eds.). Fed. Proc., Suppl. 10, p. 60–67 (1961).

Maske, H.: Über den topochemischen Nachweis von Zink im Ammonshorn verschiedener Säugetiere. Naturwissenschaften 42, 424 (1955).

Matsuba, Y., Takahashi, Y.: Spectrophotometric determination of copper with N,N,N′,N′-tetraethylthiuramdisulphide and an application of this method for studies on subcellular distribution of copper in rat brain. Analyt. Biochem. **36**, 182–191 (1970).

Maxwell, D. S., Kruger, L.: The reactive oligodendrocyte. An electron microscopic study of cerebral cortex following alpha particle irradiation. Amer. J. Anat. **118**, 437–460 (1966).

McLardy, T.: Neurosyncytial aspects of the hippocampal mossy fibre system. Confin. neurol. (Basel) **20**, 1–17 (1960).

McLardy, T.: Zinc enzymes and the hippocampal mossy fibre system. Nature (Lond.) **194**, 300–302 (1962).

McLardy, T.: Some cell and fibre peculiarities of uncal hippocampus. In: The rhinencephalon and related structures (W. Bargmann and J. P. Schadé, eds.). Progress in brain research, vol. 3, p. 71–88. Amsterdam: Elsevier 1963.

McLardy, T.: Second hippocampal zinc-rich synaptic system. Nature (Lond.) **201**, 92–93 (1964).

Mees, C. E. K., James, T. H. (eds.): The theory of the photographic process, 3rd ed. 591 pp. New York-London: Collier-Macmillan 1966.

Meessen, H., Olszewski, J.: A cytoarchitectonic atlas of the rhombencephalon of the rabbit. Basel-New York: S. Karger 1949.

Mellgren, S. I., Blackstad, T. W.: Oxidative enzymes (tetrazolium reductases) in the hippocampal region of the rat. Distribution and relation to architectonics. Z. Zellforsch. **78**, 167–207 (1967).

Mildvan, A. S.: Metals in enzyme catalysis. In: The enzymes, 3rd ed. (P. D. Boyer, ed.), vol. 2, chap. 9. New York-London: Academic Press 1970.

Morest, D. K.: Connexions of the dorsal tegmental nucleus in rat and rabbits. J. Anat. (Lond.) **95**, 229–246 (1961).

Mugnaini, E., Walberg, F., Hauglie-Hanssen, E.: Observations on the fine structure of the lateral vestibular nucleus (Deiters' nucleus) in the cat. Exp. Brain Res. **4**, 146–186 (1967).

Müller, A., Geyer, G.: Elektronenmikroskopischer Schwer-Metallnachweis in den Prosekretgranula der Panetschen Zellen. Acta histochem. (Jena) **21**, 404–405 (1965).

Müller, A., Geyer, G.: Ultrahistochemischer Metallnachweis in der Prostata der Ratte. Acta histochem. (Jena) **36**, 87–100 (1970).

Okamoto, K., Kawanishi, H.: Submicroscopic histochemical demonstration of intracellular reactive zinc in β-cells of pancreatic islets. Endocr. jap. **13**, 305–318 (1966).

O'Neal, R. M., Pla, G. W., Fox, M. R. S., Gibson, F. S., Fry, B. E.: Effect of zinc deficiency and restricted feeding on protein and ribonucleic acid metabolism of rat brain. J. Nutr. **100**, 491–497 (1970).

Pearse, A. G. E.: Histochemistry. Theoretical and applied. 3rd ed., vol. 2, chap. 28. Edinburgh-London: Churchill Livingstone 1972.

Pigache, R. M.: The anatomy of "paleocortex". A critical review. Ergebn. Anat. Entwickl.-Gesch. **43**, 6, 1–61 (1970).

Pihl, E.: Ultrastructural localization of heavy metals by a modified sulphide silver method. Histochemie **10**, 126–139 (1967).

Pihl, E., Falkmer, S.: Trials to modify the sulphide-silver method for ultrastructural tissue localization of heavy metals. Acta histochem. (Jena) **27**, 34–41 (1967).

Pletscher, A., Berneis, K. H., Da Prada, M.: A biophysical model for the storage and release of biogenic monoamines at the level of the storage organelles. In: Biochemistry of simple neuronal models (E. Costa and E. Giacobini, eds.). Advances in biochemical psychopharmacology, vol. 2, p. 205–216. New York: Raven Press 1970.

Polak, M.: Morphological and functional characteristics of the central and peripheral neuroglia (light microscopical observations). In: Biology of neuroglia (E. D. P. De Robertis and R. Carrera, eds.). Progress in brain research, vol. 15, p. 12–34. Amsterdam: Elsevier 1965.

Powell, T. P. S., Cowan, W. M.: The connexions of the midline and intralaminar nuclei of the thalamus of the rat. J. Anat. (Lond.) **88**, 307–319 (1954a).

Powell, T. P. S., Cowan, W. M.: The origin of the mamillo-thalamic tract in the rat. J. Anat. (Lond.) **88**, 489–497 (1954b).

Price, J. L., Powell, T. P. S.: An experimental study of the origin and the course of the centrifugal fibres to the olfactory bulb in the rat. J. Anat. (Lond.) **107**, 215–237 (1970).

Querido, A.: Gold intoxication of nervous elements. On the permeability of the blood-brain barrier. Acta psychiat. (Kbh.) **22**, 97–151 (1948).

Rajan, K. S., Davis, J. M., Colburn, R. W.: Metal chelates in the storage and transport of neurotransmitters: Interactions of metal ions with biogenic amines J. Neurochem. **18**, 345–364 (1971).

Rexed, B.: A cytoarchitectonic atlas of the spinal cord in the cat. J. comp. Neurol. **100**, 297–380 (1954).

Rose, J. E., Woolsey, C. N.: Structure and relations of limbic cortex and anterior thalamic nuclei in rabbit and cat. J. comp. Neurol. **89**, 279–347 (1948).

Scalia, F.: The termination of retinal axons in the pretectal region of mammals. J. comp. Neurol. **145**, 223–257 (1972).

Scheuer, P., Thorpe, M. E. C., Marriott, P.: A method for the demonstration of copper under the electron microscope. J. Histochem. Cytochem. **15**, 300–301 (1967).

Schmidt, R., Manhart, H. J.: Qualitative and quantitative Zinkbestimmung im Ammonshorn, Kleinhirn, Großhirn und Hirnstamm des Menschen. Morph. Jb. **111**, 509–514 (1968).

Siminoff, R., Schwassman, H. O., Kruger, L.: Unit analysis of the pretectal nuclear group in the rat. J. comp. Neurol. **130**, 329–342 (1967).

Spatz, H.: Über den Eisennachweis im Gehirn, besonders im Zentern des extrapyramidalmotorischen Systems. Z. ges. Neurol. Psychiat. **77**, 261–390 (1922).

Stegner, H.-E., Fischer, W.: Das Sulfidsilberverfahren zum topochemischen Schwermetallnachweis. Virchows Arch. path. Anat. **330**, 608–618 (1957).

Stensaas, L. J., Stensaas, S. S.: Astocytic neuroglial cells, oligodendrocytes and microgliacytes in the spinal cord of the toad. I. Light microscopy. Z. Zellforsch. **84**, 473–489 (1968 a).

Stensaas, L. J., Stensaas, S. S.: Astrocytic neuroglial cells, oligodendrocytes and microgliacytes in the spinal cord of the toad. II. Electron microscopy. Z. Zellforsch. **86**, 184–213 (1968 b).

Thompson, R. H. S.: The regional distribution of copper in human brain. In: Regional neurochemistry (S. S. Kety and J. Elkes, eds.), p. 102–106. Proc. Fourth Internat. Neurochem. Symposium, Varenna, 1960. Oxford: Pergamon Press 1961.

Timm, F.: Zur Histochemie des Ammonshorngebietes. Z. Zellforsch. **48**, 548–555 (1958 a).

Timm, F.: Zur Histochemie der Schwermetalle. Das Sulfid-Silber-Verfahren. Dtsch. Z. ges. gerichtl. Med. **46**, 706–711 (1958 b).

Timm, F.: Der histochemische Nachweis des Kupfers im Gehirn. Histochemie **2**, 332–341 (1961).

Timm, F.: Histochemische Lokalisation und Nachweis der Schwermetalle. Acta histochem. (Jena), Suppl. **3**, 142–148 (1962).

Timm, F., Naundorf, Ch., Kraft, M.: Zur Histochemie und Genese der chronischen Quecksilbervergiftung. Arch. Gewerbepath. Gewerbehyg. **22**, 236–245 (1966 a).

Timm, F., Neth, R.: Die normalen Schwermetalle der Niere. Histochemie **1**, 403–419 (1959).

Timm, F., Schultz, G.: Hoden und Schwermetalle. Histochemie **7**, 15–21 (1966 b).

Torvik, A., Skjörten, F.: Electron microscopic observations on nerve cell regeneration and degeneration after axon lesions. II. Changes in the glial cells. Acta neuropath. (Berl.) **17**, 265–282 (1971).

Vallee, B. L., Wacker, W. E. C.: Metalloproteins. Vol. 5 of: The proteins. Composition structure and function, 2nd ed. (H. Neurath, ed.). 192 pp. New York-London: Academic Press 1970.

Valverde, F.: Reticular formation of the albino rat's brain stem. Cytoarchitecture and corticofugal connections. J. comp. Neurol. **119**, 25–53 (1962).

Valverde, F.: The pyramidal tract in rodents. A study of its relations with the posterior column nuclei, dorsolateral reticular formation of the medulla oblongata and cervical spinal cord. (Golgi and electron microscopic observations.) Z. Zellforsch. **71**, 297–363 (1966).

Vaughn, J. E., Peters, A.: A third neuroglial cell type. An electron microscopic study. J. comp. Neurol. **133**, 269–288 (1968).

Voigt, G. E.: Histologische Versilberungen. Habil.-Schr. Jena (1951).

Voigt, G. E.: Untersuchungen mit der Sulfidsilbermethode an menschlichen und tierischen Bauchspeicheldrüsen (unter besonderer Berücksichtigung des Diabetes mellitus und experimenteller Metallvergiftungen). Virchows Arch. path. Anat. **332**, 295–323 (1959).

Voigt, G. E., Jonsson, N.: Das Sulfidsilberbild der Rattenniere bei akuten Metallsalzver-giftungen. Beitr. path. Anat. **124**, 351–360 (1961).

Weinberg, E. D.: The mutual effects of antimicrobial compounds and metallic cations. Bact. Rev. **21**, 46–68 (1957).

Welker, C.: Microelectrode delineation of fine grain somatotopic organization of SmI cerebral neocortex in albino rat. Brain Res. **26**, 259–275 (1971).

Westerfeld, W. W.: Effect of metal-binding agents on metalloproteins. In: Biological aspects of metal binding (L. A. Johnson and M. J. Seven, eds.). Fed. Proc., Suppl. **10**, 158–176 (1961).

Wong, P. Y., Fritze, K.: Determination by neutron activation of copper, manganese, and zinc in the pineal body and other areas of brain tissue. J. Neurochem. **16**, 1231–1234 (1969).

Woolsey, T. A., Loos, H. van der: The structural organization of layer IV in the somato-sensory region (SI) of mouse cerebral cortex. The description of a cortical field composed of discrete cytoarchitectonic units. Brain Res. **17**, 205–242 (1970).

Wünscher, W., Schober, W., Werner, L.: Architektonischer Atlas vom Hirnstamm der Ratte. 61 pp. Leipzig: S. Hirzel 1965.

Zemann, W., Innes, J. R. M.: Craigie's neuroanatomy of the rat. 230 pp. New York-London: Academic Press 1963.

Zimmer, J.: Ipsilateral afferents to the commissural zone of the fascia dentata, demonstrated in decommissurated rats by silver impregnation. J. comp. Neurol. **142**, 393–416 (1971).

Subject Index

Accessory olfactory bulb, see bulbus olfactorius accessorius
Amygdala 16, 31, 52
Area amygdaloidea anterior 30—31
— entorhinalis 34
— retrosplenialis e (29e) 34
— retrospleniales, see cingulate cortex
— ventralis tegmenti (Tsai) 41
Arsene 48
Axons 26, 68

Barrel field (somatosensory cortex) 32
Blood vessels 25
Boutons (see also mossy fibre boutons) 58—59
Bulbus olfactorius 27—30
— olfactorius accessorius 30

Catecholamines 61
Cerebellum 43
Cerebral cortex, see Cortex cerebri
Cerebrospinal fluid 53
Chelating agents 52, 54—55, 61—62
Choroid plexus 25
Cingulate cortex 57
Copper 61
— enzymes 62
Corpus mamillare 37, 39
— pineale 35
Cortex cerebelli, see cerebellum
Cortex cerebri, cytological distribution of staining 16
regional distribution of staining (see also individual regions) 31—34
Cranial nerve motor nuclei 42
— nerve sensory nuclei 42—43

Dendrites (see also spines) 16, 18, 58—59
Diencephalon (see also individual subdivisions and nuclei) 35—39
Diethyldithiocarbamate 52, 54, 62
2-2'-dipyridyl 54
Dithizone, behavioural effects 61
—, block of sulphide silver staining after intravital injection 52
—, intravital staining with 9, 52
—, preperfusion with (for block of sulphide silver staining) 52
Dopamine-β-hydroxylase 62
Dorsal column nuclei 42

Enzymes (see metalloenzymes)
Ependyma 25, 57

Fascia dentata, granular layer 18, 34
—, hilus (CA4) 13, 34
—, molecular layer 16, 34, 58—59

Glia 18, 21—25, 51, 56—58
—, astroglia 21, 43, 56
—, microglia 21, 27, 30, 56
—, oligoglia 21, 27, 30, 35, 56
—, perivascular glia 21—22, 24, 35, 51, 57
—, processes 18, 23, 24, 35, 57
Globus pallidus 21, 35
Grey matter (see neuropil)

Habenular nuclei 35
"Heavy metals" 48
Hippocampal region (see also individual areae)
Hippocampus, anterior continuation 31
—, field CA1 16, 34
—, field CA3 9, 16, 34
—, field CA4 34
8-hydroxyquinoline 52
Hypothalamus 18, 23, 37

Insula Calleja 30
Iron 9, 53, 61

Lamination, in cerebral cortex 58—59
Locus coeruleus 39
Lysosomes 56, 61

Medulla oblongata (see also individual nuclei) 41—43
— spinalis 43
Mesencephalon (see also individual nuclei) 16, 21, 23, 39, 41
Metal analysis (chemical and instrumental) 52, 53
— binding 52, 54, 61—62
— intoxication 51
Metalloenzymes 54, 60, 62
Mossy fibre boutons (of hippocampus) 9, 16, 34, 52, 55, 58, 61
Myelin 25—26

Neocortex 16, 32—33
Neuropil 16—18
— in the brain stem, spinal cord and cerebellum 18, 51, 59
— in the telencephalon 16, 50, 51, 58—59, 60, 61—62

Neurotransmitters 61
Nuclei accumbens 31
— caudatus-putamen 31
— centralis superior 41
— cochleares 42
— commissuralis 43
— corporis trapezoidei 18, 43
— dorsalis motorius vervi vagi 42
— dorsalis tegmenti 18, 39
— entopeduncularis 35
— habenular 35
— interpenduncularis 18, 41
— interstitialis (Cajal) 39
— lemnisci lateralis 43
— motorius nervi trigemini 42
— nervi facialis 42
— nervi hypoglossi 42
— nervi occulomotorii 42
— olfactorius anterior 30
— pontis 43
— principalis nervi trigemini 42
— reticularis tegmenti pontis 42
— ruber 41
— septal 31
— striae terminalis 31
— tractus diagonalis (Broca) 30—31
— tractus mesencephalicus nervi trigemini 41
— tractus spinalis nervi trigemini 42
— tractus solitarii 42
— ventralis tegmenti (von Gudden) 39
— vestibulares, medialis and superior 42
— vestibularis lateralis 43
— vestibularis spinalis 43

Olfactory bulb (see bulbus olfactorius)
— tubercle, see Tuberculum olfactorium
Oliva inferior 43
— superior 43
Oxine, see 8-hydroxyquinoline

Parasubiculum 34
Perikarya, neuronal 16, 51, 53, 55, 61
—, glial, see glia
Perivascular staining, see glia
Pineal body, see Corpus pineale
Pons (see also individual nuclei) 41—43
Posterior column nuclei 42
Presubiculum 34
Pretectal region 39
Proteins, see metalloproteins
Pyramidal cells of the hippocampus 18, 34
— of the neocortex 33
Pyriform cortex 16, 34

Regio preoptica laterialis 30
Reticular formation of the mesencephalon 39
— of the pons and medulla oblongata 41

Septum 31
Somata, see perikarya
Somatosensory cortex 32
Spines 58—59
Striatum, see Nucleus caudatus-putamen
Subiculum 9, 34
Substantia innominata 30
— nigra 18, 41
Substriatal grey 30
Subthalamus 37
Sulphide silver method 10—12
—, artefactual loss of staining 10, 48, 53
—, artefactual staining 10, 52—53
—, "background-browness" of neuropil 9
—, combination with other methods 12
—, electron microscopy 9, 55—56, 58
—, gum arabic 12, 50
—, paraffin embedding 10, 12, 53, 59
—, particulate nature of the precipitate 15—25, 55—56, 58
—, photography of sections 13
—, physical developer 12, 50
—, physical development 11—12, 13—14
—, "primary germs" 52
—, principles of the method 10
—, quantitative interpretation 52—55
—, selectivity 53—54, 60
—, sensitivity 53
—, solubility tests for metal sulphides 54
—, strength of development 11, 13, 50
—, sulphide treatment 10—11, 12, 48, 52
—, uniformity of staining 11
—, variability of staining 11, 50—51
Sulphydryl groups 52
Synapses 9, 59
Synaptic transmission 9, 61—62
— vesicles 58

Tanycytes 25
Telencephalon 16, 21, 50, 51, 58
Thalamus 35—37
Thiosemicarbazide 54
Transition metals 48
Tuberculum olfactorium 30

Zinc 9, 52, 61
— enzymes 60

White matter, see glia, axons, myelin